DATE DUE

RICE
in human nutrition

Prepared
in collaboration with FAO
by

Bienvenido O. Juliano
Biochemistry Unit
Plant Breeding, Genetics and Biochemistry Division
International Rice Research Institute

PUBLISHED WITH THE COLLABORATION OF
THE INTERNATIONAL RICE RESEARCH INSTITUTE

FOOD AND AGRICULTURE ORGANIZATION OF THE UNITED NATIONS
Rome, 1993

David Lubin Memorial Library Cataloguing in Publication Data

Juliano, B.O.
    Rice in human nutrition.
    (FAO Food and Nutrition Series, No. 26)
    ISBN 92-5-103149-5

    1. Rice 2. Human nutrition
    I. Title II. Series III. FAO, Rome (Italy)
    IV. International Rice Research Institute,
    Los Baños, Laguna (Philippines)

FAO code: 80   AGRIS: S01

Preface

Traditionally, rice has been the staple food and main source of income for millions of people, and it will continue to be a mainstay of life for future generations. In many countries essential development efforts are concentrated on rice to meet domestic needs for food. In the developing countries of Asia, rice is also an important item of international trade.

FAO initiated its series of nutrition studies with *Rice and rice diets: a nutrition survey*. Since its publication in 1948, our understanding of the properties of rice and rice diets has advanced significantly. In addition, enormous increases in rice production and greater sophistication in processing technology have been achieved. In response to the need to provide comprehensive and technical information reflecting these considerable changes, this new edition on rice and nutrition has been created.

The present edition is broad in scope and rich in detail. Rice cultivation practices are discussed along with patterns of rice consumption. Certain nutritional problems that are sometimes related to rice diets are described, and extensive details on the nutritional value of rice are provided. The characteristics of rice and the qualities that influence consumption and trade are covered as well as techniques for rice processing and preparation. The future of rice production in the context of concerns about population growth and the environment is discussed. An extensive bibliography is also provided.

Rice in human nutrition has been written to serve a wide range of readers in government, universities and industry as a general source on most aspects of rice production, processing, trade and consumption. We hope that this book, as well as complementary trade information on rice published by FAO, will successfully address many readers' questions about this important food and assist in development and training activities in all countries.

John R. Lupien
Director
Food Policy and Nutrition Division

Contents

Chapter 1
Introduction

Rice (*Oryza sativa* L.) is the most important cereal crop in the developing world and is the staple food of over half the world's population. It is generally considered a semi-aquatic annual grass plant. About 20 species of the genus *Oryza* are recognized, but nearly all cultivated rice is *O. sativa* L. A small amount of *Oryza glaberrima*, a perennial species, is grown in Africa. So-called "wild rice" (*Zizania aquatica*), grown in the Great Lakes region of the United States, is more closely related to oats than to rice.

Because of its long history of cultivation and selection under diverse environments, *O. sativa* has acquired a broad range of adaptability and tolerance so that it can be grown in a wide range of water/soil regimens from deeply flooded land to dry hilly slopes (Lu and Chang, 1980). In Asia, cultivars with resistance to aluminum toxicity and with tolerance to submergence by flood water (IRRI, 1975), (Figure 1), high salinity and cool temperatures at the seedling or ripening stage have been developed (Chang, 1983). In Africa, cultivars with tolerance to iron toxicity and heat constraints have also been developed and cultivated. Rice is now grown in over 100 countries on every continent except Antarctica, extending from 50° north latitude to 40° south latitude and from sea level to an altitude of 3 000 m.

ORIGIN AND SPREAD OF RICE

The geographical site of the origin of rice domestication is not yet definitely known. The general consensus is that rice domestication occurred independently in China, India and Indonesia, thereby giving rise to three races of rice: sinica (also known as japonica), indica and javanica (also known as bulu in Indonesia). There are indications that rice was cultivated in India between 1500 and 2000 B.C. and in Indonesia around 1648 B.C. Archaeological findings have shown that tropical or indica rice was being cultivated in Ho-mu-tu, Chekiang Province, China at least 7 000 years ago (Chang, 1983). Recently, remains of the temperate or sinica (japonica) rice of the same age were found at Lou-jia-jiao, also in Chekiang Province (Chang, 1985). Rice was rapidly dispersed from its tropical (southern and southeastern Asia) and subtropical (southwestern and southern China) habitats to much higher altitudes and latitudes in Asia, reaching Japan as recently as 2 300 years ago (Chang, 1983). It was introduced to points as far as West Africa, North America and Australia within the last six centuries.

FIGURE 1
The world's rice land classified by water regimes and predominant rice type

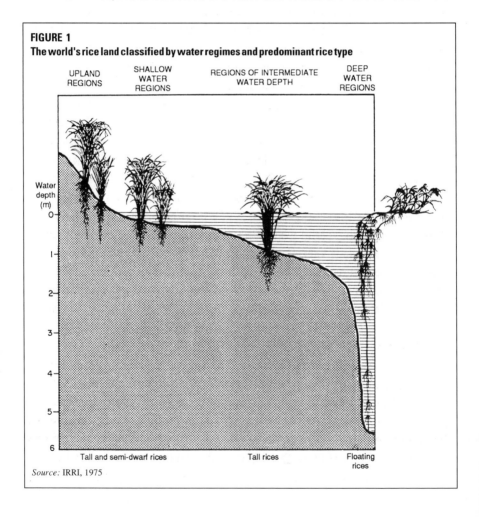

UPLAND REGIONS   SHALLOW WATER REGIONS   REGIONS OF INTERMEDIATE WATER DEPTH   DEEP WATER REGIONS

Water depth (m)

Tall and semi-dwarf rices   Tall rices   Floating rices

Source: IRRI, 1975

Rice growing became firmly established in South Carolina in the United States in about 1690 (Adair, 1972). Rice was cultivated in Europe from the eighth century in Portugal and Spain and by the ninth to the tenth century in southern Italy (Lu and Chang, 1980).

WORLD RICE PRODUCTION COMPARED TO OTHER CEREALS

The world annual cereal production for 1989 is shown in Table 1. About 95 percent of the world's rice is produced in developing countries and 92 percent of it in Asia. In contrast only about 42 percent of the wheat produced is grown in developing countries. Production of rice, exports and imports and estimated irrigated areas of major rice producing countries are shown in Table 2. In 1988, China was the principal rice producer (35 percent) followed by India (22 percent), Indonesia (8.5 percent), Bangladesh (4.7 percent), Thailand (4.3 percent) and Viet Nam (3.4 percent). Of the major rice producers only Pakistan, the United States and Egypt had 100 percent irrigated rice land (IRRI, 1991a). Non-irrigated rice cultivation predominates in many countries, such as Thailand and Brazil.

Among the cereals, rice production uses the highest proportion of land area. Of the 147.5 million ha of land devoted to rice production worldwide in 1989, developing countries contributed 141.4 million ha, or 96 percent. Asia accounted for 90 percent of the world's land area cultivated to rice; in this region, 132.1 million ha are used for this crop (FAO, 1990a).

Mean yields of cereal crops in various regions of the world in 1989 were lower in developing countries than in developed countries (FAO, 1990a), (Table 3). Rough rice yields were highest in Oceania, mainly Australia, followed by Europe and North and Central America, and were lowest in Africa and South America.

When the yields of the various cereals were adjusted using conversion factors based on extraction rates, rice was shown to have the highest food yield among the cereals (Table 4). Food energy yields were approximately proportional to food yields, since energy contents of the cereals are similar. Food protein yield, however, was higher in white wheat flour than in milled rice because the protein content of wheat flour is higher than that of milled rice.

TABLE 1
Annual production of cereal crops, total tubers and roots and pulses by region, 1989 (million tonnes)

Region	Wheat	Rough rice	Maize	Sorghum	Millet	Barley	Rye	Oats	Total cereals	Total tubers and roots	Soybean, peanut and pulses
Africa	12.7	10.7	37.0	13.7	9.3	5.6	0.01	0.2	90.5	102.6	11.7
North and Central America	84.2	9.5	212.0	22.0	0.2	20.9	1.2	9.1	360.6	23.8	59.9
South America	19.0	17.1	36.6	3.1	0.05	1.2	0.1	1.1	78.4	43.7	36.3
Asia	192.0	469.9	113.7	19.1	15.2	15.3	1.2	0.9	830.0	242.0	55.4
Europe	127.5	2.2	55.5	0.6	0.03	71.6	13.5	11.7	290.9	103.0	10.1
Oceania	14.3	0.8	0.3	1.2	0.02	4.4	0.02	1.7	23.0	2.9	1.8
Soviet Union	92.3	2.6	15.3	0.2	4.1	48.5	20.1	16.8	201.3	72.0	12.5
World	542.0	512.7	470.5	59.9	28.9	167.6	36.1	41.6	1 874.7	590.2	185.6
Developed countries	317.2	25.5	280.8	18.1	4.3	145.7	34.8	39.3	877.1	203.6	80.4
Developing countries	224.7	487.2	189.7	41.8	24.6	21.9	1.3	2.3	997.6	386.6	105.2

Sources: FAO, 1990a, 1990b.

TABLE 2
Rough rice production and rice imports and exports, 1988, and estimated irrigated rice area, 1987

Region or country	Rough rice production (*million tonnes*)	Rice imports[a] (*million tonnes*)	Rice exports[a] (*million tonnes*)	Irrigated area (*% of rice area*)
World	492 137	11 408	12 185	53
Asia	449 252	5 309	8 099	
Bangladesh	23 097	674	–	19
China	173 515	314	802	93
Hong Kong	–	364	12	–
India	106 385	684	350	44
Indonesia	41 676	33	–	81
Iraq	141	603	–	–
Japan	12 419	16	–	99
Korea, DPR	5 400	–	200	67
Korea, Rep. of	8 260	1	1	99
Malaysia	1 783	284	5	54
Myanmar	13 164	–	64	18
Pakistan	4 800	–	1 210	100
Philippines	8 971	119	–	58
Saudi Arabia	–	363	–	–
Singapore	–	213	3	–
Sri Lanka	2 477	194	–	77
Thailand	21 263	–	5 267	27
Viet Nam	17 000	176	97	46
North and Central America	9 509	699	2 261	
United States	7 253	0	2 260	100
Africa	9 785	2 589	87	
Egypt	2 132	–	71	100

(continued)

TABLE 2 (continued)

Region or country	Rough rice production (*million tonnes*)	Rice imports[a] (*million tonnes*)	Rice exports[a] (*million tonnes*)	Irrigated area (*% of rice area*)
Madagascar	2 149	37	0	31
Nigeria	1 400	200	0	16
South America	17 741	255	467	
Brazil	11 806	108	26	18
Europe	2 211	1 827	950	
Italy	1 093	95	510	
Australia	740	0	297	
Soviet Union	2 866	498	22	

[a]Milled rice basis. Conversion factor from rough rice to milled rice is 0.7.
Sources: FAO, 1990a; IRRI, 1991a.

TABLE 3
Mean yield of cereal crops by region, 1989 (t/ha)

Region	Wheat	Rough rice	Maize	Sorghum	Millet	Barley	Rye	Oats	Total cereals
Africa	1.47	1.95	1.77	0.81	0.65	1.12	0.13	0.21	1.22
North and Central America	2.10	5.09	5.92	3.37	1.20	2.52	1.79	1.83	3.65
South America	1.90	2.50	2.10	2.23	1.11	1.71	1.02	1.45	2.09
Asia	2.32	3.56	2.90	1.04	0.77	1.41	1.44	1.51	2.71
Europe	4.60	5.35	4.96	3.74	1.22	4.04	3.03	2.89	4.26
Oceania	1.59	7.40	4.93	1.86	0.89	1.80	0.54	1.48	1.69
Soviet Union	1.94	3.90	3.72	1.22	1.48	1.76	1.87	1.56	1.90
World	2.40	3.48	3.66	1.35	0.78	2.31	2.14	1.79	2.66
Developed countries	2.53	5.86	6.05	3.17	1.46	2.60	2.18	1.83	3.10
Developing countries	2.24	3.40	2.31	1.08	0.72	1.32	1.40	1.36	2.37

Source: FAO, 1990a.

TABLE 4

Comparison of grain yield, food energy yield and protein yield of cereals based on energy and protein contents and conversion factor (extraction rate)

Cereal	Mean yield (t/ha)	Conversion factor	Conversion factor derivation	Adjusted yield (t/ha)	Energy content (kcal/g)	Food energy yield (10⁻⁶ kcal/g)	Protein content[a] (%)	Adjusted protein (%N x 6.25)	Food protein yield (t/ha)
Wheat	2.40	0.73	white flour	1.8	3.85	6.9	11.2	12.3	0.22
Rough rice	3.48	0.70	milled rice	2.4	3.75	9.0	7.5	7.9	0.19
Maize	3.66	0.56	corn meal	2.0	3.97	7.9	7.5	7.5	0.15
Sorghum	1.35	0.80	white flour	1.1	3.85	4.2	8.3	8.3	0.09
Millet	0.78	1.0	whole grain	0.78	3.94	3.1	5.6	5.6	0.04
Barley	2.31	0.55	white flour	1.3	3.90	5.1	8.2	8.2	0.11
Rye	2.14	0.83	white flour	1.8	3.75	6.8	7.3	8.0	0.14
Oats	1.79	0.58	white oats	1.0	3.92	3.9	14.2	14.2	0.14

[a] N factor was 6.25, except 5.7 for wheat and rye and 5.95 for rice.
Sources: FAO, 1990a; Lu & Chang, 1980; Eggum, 1969, 1977, 1979.

METHODS OF RICE PRODUCTION

Irrigated rice

Review of rice production methods has shown that practices range from very primitive to highly mechanized (De Datta, 1981; Luh, 1980; Yoshida, 1981). Tractors and two-wheeled power tillers are the most important agricultural machines used for rice production (Barker, Herdt and Rose, 1985). In 1980 the number of power tillers used per 1 000 ha was from 0.1 to 26 in tropical Asia, 56 in China, 73 in Taiwan (province of China), 198 in the Republic of Korea and 1 158 in Japan. In Asia, animals (buffalo and water buffalo, carabao) are still used for ploughing and harrowing. Land preparation may be carried out while the soil is dry or wet, depending on the water supply. For irrigated rice, the soil is prepared wet or puddled in Asia, but puddling is not generally practiced in America, Europe and Africa. In areas without a hard pan, where animals and tractors sink in the mud, the soil is prepared with hand hoes. Regardless of whether the land is prepared wet or dry, the water is always held on the lowland fields by bunds.

Most irrigated rice is transplanted, although direct seeding is becoming more extensive. The seeds are pregerminated and grown in wet seed-beds for 9 to 14, 20 to 25 or 40 to 50 days after sowing and are then transplanted either by hand or by mechanical transplanters. The number of seedlings per hill may vary from one to eight. Direct seeding is done by broadcasting the pregerminated grain by hand in Asia or by water-seeding by airplane in the United States and Australia. The seeds may also be machine-drilled in

Rice ploughing with buffaloes

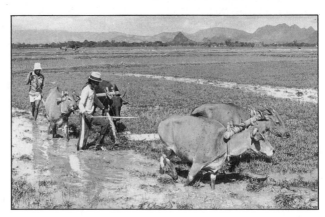

puddled soil or drill-seeded into dry soil. Deep-water rice is commonly dry-seeded, but it is occasionally transplanted or double transplanted.

Ideally, water is maintained in the rice field to suppress weed growth during the growing season. Hand weeding and mechanical or rotary weeders are popular. Herbicides are also economical and effective. Fertilization is normally practised for increased yield, particularly with the modern, semi-dwarf or high-yielding varieties which respond well to fertilizer without lodging. Both inorganic and organic fertilizers are used, including green manures such as the leguminous shrub *Sesbania* spp. and the water plants *Azolla* and *Anabaena* spp. Modern rice varieties increase in grain yield by 6 kg per kg of applied fertilizer in the wet season and by 9 kg per kg of applied fertilizer in the dry season. Total fertilizer nutrients range from 10 to 100 kg/ha in tropical Asia and from 200 to 350 kg/ha in Japan, Taiwan and the Republic of Korea (Barker, Herdt and Rose, 1985).

Other rice ecosystems
Rain-fed lowland rice is grown on puddled soil in fields bounded by dykes that can pond water to depths of 0 to 25 cm (shallow) and 25 to 50 cm (medium), depths seldom exceeded in such areas (Huke and Huke, 1990). The irrigation water is not received from river diversions, storage reservoirs or deep wells, but from rainfall or runoff from a local catchment area. The prevailing climatic and soil conditions in shallow rain-fed rice areas are extremely variable. In deep-water (50 to 100 cm) rain-fed lowland rice, modern semi-dwarf varieties cannot be used. Fertilizer use is low, stand establishment difficult and pest control almost impossible, and yields are poor. Rain-fed lowland rice is next to irrigated rice in importance in terms of harvested area and production of rice (Table 5).

Upland rice is grown in fields that are not bunded but are prepared and seeded under dry conditions and depend on rainfall for moisture (Huke and Huke, 1990). In Brazil, a major part of the rice crop is upland. In India and throughout Southeast Asia, upland cultivation is common along river banks as waters recede at the end of the rainy season. Soils are commonly heavy and residual moisture alone sustains growth. Upland rice farming ranges from shifting cultivation of forested hilly or mountainous areas that are

TABLE 5

Harvested area, yield and rough rice production in 37 major rice-producing developing countries, by ecosystem, 1985

Ecosystem	Area		Yield (t/ha)	Production	
	(million ha)	(%)		(million t)	(%)
Irrigated	67	49	4.7	313	72
Rain-fed lowland	40	29	2.1	84	19
Upland	18	13	1.1	21	5
Deep-water/tidal wetland	13	9	1.5	19	4
Total	138	100	3.2[a]	437	100

[a]Weighted average.
Source: IRRI, 1989.

cleared and burned to large-scale mechanized operations. Between these two extremes is farming of sloping hill regions that are subject to serious erosion and frequent drought, by hundreds of thousands of the poorest of rice farmers. The environmental damage here is very serious. In South and Southeast Asia some 13 percent of the total rice area is upland, but in some countries in Africa and Latin America upland rice exceeds 50 percent of the national total rice area. Yields are lowest in upland rice (Table 5).

In deep-water rice, water depth is at least 1 m during a significant portion of the growing season. In large parts of Bangladesh as well as in portions of the Mekong and the Chao Praya Deltas, water depth may exceed 5 m, but it is normally between 1 and 3 m in other regions (Huke and Huke, 1990). Where water rises rapidly after the start of the monsoon rains, rice is commonly broadcast in unpuddled fields that are seldom bounded by dykes of any sort. The varieties planted are tall and leafy, with few tillers. They are photoperiod sensitive and mature only after the rainy season. They can elongate and float as the water level rises. Major dyking and flood control projects in the last two decades have upgraded many former deep-water rice areas into the rain-fed or irrigated category in Bangladesh, India, Thailand and southern Viet Nam.

HARVESTING

Tropical rice is usually harvested at 20 percent or more moisture about 30 days after 50 percent flowering, when grains will provide optimum total and head rice yields. Moisture content at harvest is lower during the dry season than in the wet season because of sun-drying while the grains are in the intact plant. The actual period of dry-matter production is no more than 14 to 18 days, after which the grain undergoes drying.

Harvesting is carried out by cutting the stem, sun-drying and then threshing by hand by beating the rice heads on a slotted bamboo platform, by having animals or people tread on the crop or by the use of mechanical threshers. Combine harvesters are used in large areas such as the Muda estate in Malaysia and in the United States, Australia, Europe and Latin America.

Sun-drying to 14 percent moisture is a common practice but is unreliable during the wet season. Many mechanical dryers have been designed but have not been popular with farmers and processors. After drying, the rough rice is winnowed to remove the chaff using either a hand winnower or a manually operated wooden winnower.

LABOUR USE

More labour may be used by Asian farmers growing modern varieties than by those growing traditional varieties (Barker, Herdt & Rose, 1985). The contribution of family labour and hired labour is quite variable with location.

The various steps in rice cultivation include seed selection, seed-bed and land preparation, transplanting, weeding, fertilizing, pest management, harvesting, threshing, drying and marketing. Huke and Huke (1990) estimated that the labour requirements for one hectare of low-intensity rice production relying on rainfall for water and using improved IR36 seed and 50 kg of urea fertilizer are about 84 person-days and 14 animal-days to yield 2.5 tonnes of rough rice. In obtaining the 2.5 tonne yield, harvesting with a sickle and hand threshing against a log will consume at least 22 person-days. By contrast, labour input in high-technology California rice production of about 350 ha is 40 person-days (Herdt, 1986).

Huke and Huke (1990) calculated the energy efficiency of low-intensity rice production at a specific site in the Philippines to be 12 calories per calorie expended. Under medium and high inputs, output ratios were 7 to 8 calories per calorie expended.

While women make up 25 to 70 percent of the labour in rice farming systems in Asia, their role has not been recognized until recently and their needs have remained unaddressed in technology development (Feldstein and Poats, 1990). They participate in rice and rice-related production, marketing and processing activities. It is now widely appreciated that women are often active in agricultural production and that they, as well as men, are potential users and beneficiaries of new technology. Gender analysis is now integrated into research projects and priority is given to technologies that reduce the burden of rural women without displacing their income-generating capacities. These technologies include integrated pest management, seed management and post-harvest rice utilization and processing (Unnevehr and Stanford, 1985).

PRODUCTION COSTS

The total cost of producing one tonne of rough rice in 1987-89 is compared for irrigated upland and rain-fed rice in Table 6. Total cost per hectare and grain yield were highest for irrigated rice and lowest for upland rice.

MODERN HIGH-YIELD VARIETIES

In the 1950s, growth in rice production in most Asian countries was due to expansion of the area planted, but in the 1960s and 1970s yield increase was more important (Barker, Herdt and Rose, 1985). Contributing factors were the introduction of semi-dwarf varieties and higher fertilizer inputs.

The semi-dwarf varieties developed at the International Rice Research Institute (IRRI) have a plant type that contrasts with that of the tall, traditional, photoperiod-sensitive varieties. They have erect leaves, are heavy tillering and have low photoperiod sensitivity. Their plant architecture allows them to absorb nutrients without lodging and allows sunlight to penetrate the leaf canopy. Growth duration is shorter in the modern varieties and is close to 100 days from seeding, which allow three crops per year. At

TABLE 6
Cost of producing one tonne of rough rice, 1987-89 (US$)

Country	Irrigated	Upland	Rain-fed
Argentina	870	–	–
Colombia	204	–	194
Ecuador	441	196	295
India	–	–	303
Indonesia	82	141	104
Italy	543	–	–
Japan	3 676	–	–
Korea, Republic of	939	–	–
Nepal	96	–	108
Philippines	124	–	–
Portugal	376	–	–
Thailand	98	–	–
United States	481	–	–

Source: FAO, 1991.

low input levels, they yield comparably to traditional varieties. However, in all cases, modern varieties outperform traditional varieties, given additional inputs of energy, insecticides and fertilizers.

By 1981-84, modern varieties covered 13 percent of the total rice area in Thailand, 34 percent in the Republic of Korea, 25 percent in China, 25 percent in Bangladesh, 36 percent in Nepal, 54 percent in Malaysia, 46 percent in Pakistan, 49 percent in Myanmar, 54 percent in India, 82 percent in Indonesia, 85 percent in the Philippines and 87 percent in Sri Lanka (Dalrymple, 1986). The low adoption rate in Thailand is due to the requirement in that country for long-grain varieties (brown rice length greater than 7 mm) for export. More than 60 percent of the world's rice area is now planted to varieties of improved plant type.

The yield potentials of the new modern varieties are no better than those of the first modern variety, IR8, but they show improved resistance to insect pests and diseases and increased tolerance to environmental stresses. However, their increased resistances are single-gene characteristics which are overcome by the pests in a few years. Insect resurgence has been documented in which insecticide spraying increased the insect population instead of reducing it (Chelliah and Heinrichs, 1984). Alternative approaches of horizontal or multiline resistance are considered necessary, as there is a rapid breakdown of resistance to the brown planthopper because of the appearance of new insect biotypes. No source of resistance to tungro virus disease has been identified in cultivated rice, *O. sativa*. However, resistance sources have been identified in wild species and are being introduced through wide crosses to *O. sativa*.

FARM UNITS

The mean size of the rice farm is less than 1 ha in Bangladesh, Japan, the Republic of Korea and Sri Lanka, over 1 ha in Indonesia and Nepal, about 2 ha in Malaysia, Pakistan and the Philippines and about 3 ha in Thailand (IRRI, 1991a). The most common types of tenure are share-cropping and fixed rent (Barker, Herdt and Rose, 1985). Share-cropping is widely practised in Bangladesh, India, Pakistan and Indonesia. Fixed-rent systems exist in all countries of the region, but are less common than share rents. In land reform in China, North Korea, Viet Nam and Myanmar, land has been expropriated by governments and held in public ownership; in Japan and Taiwan, former tenants were deemed owners. In the Philippines, the 1972 land reform for fixed-rent tenants was rapidly implemented, but land ownership transfer has been slow.

RICE TRADE

About 4 percent of the world's rice production enters international trade. The major exporters in 1988 were Thailand, the United States and Pakistan, while the major importers were Iraq, the Soviet Union, Hong Kong, Saudi Arabia, Malaysia, Singapore, Sri Lanka, Nigeria, Bangladesh and Brazil (FAO, 1990a, Table 2). Viet Nam became the third largest rice exporter in the world in 1989, with 1.38 million metric tons of milled rice (IRRI, 1991a).

PESTS AND DISEASES

Pests and diseases are major problems in the tropics, particularly with rice monoculture, since hosts are continuously present in the environment. Rodents, birds and golden snails all reduce rice yields. The major insect pests are the yellow stem borer, the green leafhopper, which is the vector of the tungro virus, and brown planthoppers, which cause hopperburn. Insect control has been attempted by breeding varieties with improved resistance to the pests. Integrated pest management is becoming more popular in view of the problem of insect resurgence from the excessive use of insecticides.

The major diseases of rice plants in tropical Asia remain the rice blast fungus and bacterial leaf blight. The existence of many races of the blast fungus makes control difficult. Blast is a particular problem in upland rice. The major virus disease is the tungro virus, transmitted by the green leafhopper. The rice weevil and hoja blanca are the main problems in Latin America, while yellow mottle virus and diopsis predominate in Africa.

The incorporation of resistance into rice varieties is complicated by the presence of many races of diseases, as in blast, and the existence of biotypes of pests, as in the brown planthopper.

CONCLUSION

The great production gains in the 1960s and 1970s occurred in the irrigated and favourable rain-fed lowland areas, where short-duration, semi-dwarf varieties could express their high yield potential. Mean farm yields of irrigated rice in many countries are still about 3 to 5 tonnes per ha, but some farmers can obtain twice that. Irrigated land now comprises about half of total harvested area, but it contributes more than two-thirds of total production and is expected to continue to dominate the sector (Table 5). The less favourable environments (unfavourable rain-fed lowland, upland, and deep-water and tidal wetland) produce 20 to 25 percent of the world's rice. These rice ecosystems must sustain farmers and consumers who so far have received little benefit from modern advances in rice technology.

Chapter 2

Rice consumption
and nutrition problems
in rice-consuming countries

In 39 countries rice is the staple diet, but the dependence on rice for food energy is much higher in Asia than in other regions (FAO, 1984), (Table 7). The energy dependence on rice in South and Southeast Asia is higher than the energy dependence on any other staples in other regions. South Asia also has the lowest energy intake. Rice provides 35 to 59 percent of energy consumed for 2 700 million people in Asia (FAO, 1984). A mean of 8 percent of food energy is supplied by rice for 1 000 million people in Africa and Latin America.

FAO statistics for 1987-89 showed that rice availability per caput could supply from 19 to over 76 percent of total food energy in different Asian countries (Table 8). This range is equivalent to a milled rice availability ranging from 40 to 161 kg per caput annually.

The contribution of rice to protein in the diet, based on FAO *Food balance sheets* for 1979-81, was 69.2 percent in South Asia and 51.4 percent in Southeast Asia (FAO, 1984), (Table 7). These percentages are higher than the contribution of any other cereal protein in any region of the world.

With the exception of the highest income countries in Asia, per caput rice consumption has remained stable or has increased moderately over the past 30 years. Total consumption continues to increase in close association with population and income growth. Rice supply, personal income and the availability and price of dietary substitutes are key determinants of the diversity in Asian diets, in addition to the quality of the rice being consumed. The greatest factor affecting demand, however, continues to be the unabated

TABLE 7

Energy and protein contribution to diets in developing-country regions by commodity, 1979-81

Region	Energy contribution (% of regional total)						Total energy (kcal/day)	Protein contribution (% of regional total)		
	Rice	Wheat	Maize	Barley	Sorghum and millet	Roots, tubers and plantain		Rice	Other cereals	Roots, tubers and plantain
Temperate South America[a]	1.3	30.7	1.4	0.2	0	4.7	3 178	1.0	20.4	2.4
Tropical South America[b]	14.9	12.8	9.3	0.3	0	11.9	2 514	12.9	19.7	3.6
Central America[c]	5.1	11.4	35.0	0	0.6	4.0	2 655	5.0	37.4	0
East/Southern Africa[d]	3.0	5.7	33.6	0	4.6	23.0	2 047	2.9	48.1	5.9
Equatorial Africa[e]	9.5	2.3	8.4	0.1	5.9	46.4	2 153	11.8	30.0	12.9
Humid West Africa[f]	18.3	4.5	10.6	–	4.1	35.2	2 120	20.3	20.2	15.9
Semi-arid West Africa[g]	6.8	4.6	5.6	0.1	31.1	20.9	2 290	6.9	42.7	9.7
North Africa/Near East[h]	6.0	39.6	5.8	2.6	4.5	1.7	2 594	5.1	53.0	0.9

(continued)

TABLE 7 (continued)

Region	Energy contribution (% of regional total)						Total energy (kcal/day)	Protein contribution (% of regional total)		
	Rice	Wheat	Maize	Barley	Sorghum and millet	Roots, tubers and plantain		Rice	Other cereals	Roots, tubers and plantain
India	33.2	18.5	3.1	0.7	11.0	2.5	2 056	32.3	35.4	0
South Asia[i]	68.0	9.9	2.5	0.1	0.4	3.7	1 898	69.2	13.1	0
Southeast Asia[i]	56.1	4.7	6.1	0.6	0.4	7.6	2 414	51.4	10.1	1.4
China	35.4	18.4	7.7	0.6	2.9	12.1	2 428	28.6	26.9	5.0
All developing countries	29.3	17.5	7.6	0.8	4.9	9.1	2 349	25.3	29.1	2.7

[a] Argentina, Chile, Uruguay.
[b] Bolivia, Brazil, Colombia, Ecuador, Guyana, Paraguay, Peru, Suriname, Venezuela.
[c] Costa Rica, Cuba, the Dominican Republic, El Salvador, Guatemala, Haiti, Honduras, Mexico, Nicaragua.
[d] Angola, Botswana, Kenya, Lesotho, Malawi, Mozambique, Swaziland, United Republic of Tanzania, Zambia, Zimbabwe.
[e] Burundi, Cameroon, the Central African Republic, the Congo, Gabon, Madagascar, Rwanda, Uganda, Zaire.
[f] Benin, Côte d'Ivoire, Ghana, Guinea, Liberia, Sierra Leone, Togo.
[g] Burkina Faso, Chad, the Gambia, Guinea-Bissau, Mali, Mauritania, the Niger, Nigeria, Senegal.
[h] Afghanistan, Algeria, Cyprus, Egypt, Ethiopia, Islamic Republic of Iran, Iraq, Jordan, Lebanon, the Libyan Arab Jamahiriya, Morocco, Pakistan, Saudi Arabia, Somalia, the Sudan, the Syrian Arab Republic, Tunisia, Turkey, Yemen AR, Yemen PDR.
[i] Bangladesh, Nepal, Sri Lanka.
[j] Bhutan, Cambodia, Indonesia, Democratic People's Republic of Korea, Republic of Korea, Laos, Malaysia, Myanmar, the Philippines, Thailand, Viet Nam.
Source: FAO, 1984.

TABLE 8
Per caput availability of milled rice and contribution of rice to dietary energy and protein in selected rice-eating countries

Country	Availability of milled rice (*kg/caput/year*)	% Contribution of rice	
		Energy	Protein
Bangladesh	142	73	63
Belize	25	9	7
Brazil	41	16	14
Brunei	94	36	23
Cambodia	173	80	71
China	104	38	27
Colombia	36	25	13
Comoros	78	42	37
Côte d'Ivoire	63	23	22
Dominican Republic	44	19	18
Gambia	98	40	32
Guinea	59	28	26
Guinea-Bissau	116	48	45
Guyana	86	33	29
Hong Kong	59	21	12
India	68	31	24
Indonesia	140	59	49
Japan	64	25	14
Korea, DPR	125	48	29
Korea, Republic of	98	38	25
Liberia	110	43	49
Madagascar	111	53	50
Malaysia	84	31	26
Maldives	60	26	14
Mauritius	71	26	16
Myanmar	187	76	68

(continued)

TABLE 8 (continued)

Country	Availability of milled rice (*kg/caput/year*)	% Contribution of rice	
		Energy	Protein
Nepal	94	44	35
Papua New Guinea	39	16	14
Philippines	92	40	31
Seychelles	68	30	21
Sierra Leone	89	44	41
Singapore	58	19	12
Sri Lanka	92	42	39
Suriname	103	35	30
Thailand	132	58	48
Vanuatu	43	17	12
Viet Nam	147	68	62

Source: FAO (Statistics Division), 1987-89 average, except China, which is 1984-86 average.

population growth, particularly in the poorest countries wherein rice constitutes the most important component of the diet (Huang, 1987).

Within a country, rice consumption is higher in the rural than in the urban areas. While income elasticity for rice will undoubtedly decline as income increases, only Japan, Malaysia, Singapore, Taiwan and Thailand have income levels that support negative estimates of income elasticities for rice (Huang, David and Duff, 1991), (Table 9). However, the population and rice consumption of these five countries account for less than 10 percent of totals for Asia. In most Asian countries, therefore, rice is not an inferior food and income elasticities for rice will likely remain positive throughout the 1990s.

NUTRITIONAL PROBLEMS IN RICE-CONSUMING COUNTRIES

The nutritional situation in rice-consuming countries varies substantially depending on a web of interacting socio-economic, developmental, cultural, environmental and dietary factors. Regardless of the region, most rice-dependent economies have high population growth rates, low rice yields

TABLE 9

Key indicators of developing Asian countries, rough rice yield and income elasticity for rice

Country	Economically active population, 1985 (%)	Percent agriculture in economically active population, 1985	Cropped land per caput, 1985 (ha)	Literacy rate, 1985 (%)	Life expectancy at birth, 1985 (yr)	Per caput GNP, 1987 (US$)	Rough rice yield, 1988 (t/ha)	Income elasticity for rice, 1988[a]
Afghanistan	30.1	57.9	0.49	23	(37)	–	2.29	
Bangladesh	28.5	71.8	0.09	33	51	160	2.36	0.125
Bhutan	44.6	91.6	0.07	(10)[b]	44	–	1.66	
Cambodia	49.5	72.3	0.42	(66)	–	–	1.33	
China	–	–	0.00	(59)	69	300	5.35	0.299
Hong Kong	51.7	1.6	0.00	88	76	8 260	–	
India	38.6	68.1	0.22	43	57	300	2.54	0.237
Indonesia	38.1	52.8	0.13	74	55	450	4.11	0.446
Korea, Republic of	40.7	30.1	0.05	(96)	69	2 690	6.56	0.174
Laos	48.9	73.7	0.22	84	45	–	1.91	
Malaysia	39.7	36.7	0.28	73	70	1 800	2.68	–0.349

(continued)

TABLE 9 (continued)

Country	Economically active population, 1985 (%)	Percent agriculture in economically active population, 1985	Cropped land per caput, 1985 (ha)	Literacy rate, 1985 (%)	Life expectancy at birth, 1985 (yr)	Per caput GNP, 1987 (US$)	Rough rice yield, 1988 (t/ha)	Income elasticity for rice, 1988[a]
Myanmar	44.9	50.0	0.27	81	59	–	2.26	0.524
Nepal	41.7	92.4	0.14	25	47	160	2.26	0.435
Pakistan	29.7	52.1	0.20	29	51	350	2.35	0.324
Philippines	36.5	49.2	0.14	86	63	590	2.64	0.522
Singapore	47.9	1.3	0.00	86	73	7 940	–	
Sri Lanka	36.5	52.5	0.14	87	70	400	3.04	
Taiwan, Province of China	–	–	–	92	73	–	4.86	–0.591
Thailand	51.9	67.7	0.38	91	64	840	2.15	–0.328
Viet Nam	48.2	64.1	0.11	(84)	65	–	2.97	

[a] Japan, –0.530.
[b] Figures in parentheses are 1980 values.
Sources: Asian Development Bank, 1989; IRRI, 1991a (rough rice yield); Huang, David and Duff, 1991 (income elasticity).

(except for China, Korea and Indonesia) and low gross national product (IRRI, 1989), (Table 9). Landholdings are small, low percentages of the population are economically active and literacy rates are variable in tropical Asia (Asian Development Bank, 1989), (Table 9).

Malnutrition is not just a problem of food availability; it is also a problem of income and food and income distribution (Flinn and Unnevehr, 1984). Because rice is a major source of income in rural Asia as well as a key component of private expenditure, increased productivity can reduce malnutrition both by increasing the incomes of the poorest rice producers and by increasing the availability of rice and the stability of rice prices.

A summary of nutritional problems prevalent in rice-consuming countries is presented. As 90 percent of the rice is produced and eaten by populations in Southeast Asia, the description is biased toward that region.

Among the major nutritional problems prevalent in rice-consuming countries, inadequate and unbalanced dietary intake is the most important one. In combination with other compounding factors, it leads to widespread prevalence of protein-energy malnutrition (PEM), nutritional anaemia (particularly from iron deficiency), vitamin A deficiency and iodine deficiency disorders (Chong, 1979; Scrimshaw, 1988; Khor, Tee and Kandiah, 1990). In addition, dietary deficiencies of thiamine, riboflavin, calcium, vitamin C and zinc are prevalent in many areas but often are not manifested in overt clinical syndromes.

These nutritional problems are not caused directly by the consumption of rice *per se* but reflect an overall impact of multiple causative factors similar to those of other developing countries where rice is not a major staple.

Food availability and dietary intake

Data on availability of food and nutrients are derived from FAO *Food balance sheets* and from nutrition surveys and studies on food consumption.

Food balance sheet data provide estimates of per caput food and nutrient availability taking into consideration food production, imports, exports, non-food uses, manufactured foods and wastage at the retail level. A comparison of daily nutrient supply for developed and developing countries (FAO, 1990b), (Table 10) shows that the Far East has the lowest availability of fat, retinol, thiamine, riboflavin and ascorbic acid. Individual data pertaining to rice-eating countries (Table 11) show that in addition to dietary energy many rice-consuming countries have unsatisfactory levels of fat, calcium, iron, riboflavin and ascorbic acid. When wastage at the household level, including cooking loss, is taken into account the supply situation becomes more precarious.

Available data from nutrition surveys are often fragmentary and do not pertain to all countries. Even when data are available they may not always be representative and are often out of date. Table 12 presents examples of available data on average consumption of energy and protein from selected countries. Overall this consumption is unsatisfactory when compared with availability of these nutrients, except in China and Mauritius (Table 11). There appears to be a large gap between availability of food and actual consumption, which indicates a significant influence of factors related to food access and utilization. However, these intake values strongly suggest the possibility of widespread prevalence of protein-energy malnutrition in young children. There is also enough indication from available consumption studies to suggest that special groups such as young children and pregnant mothers have dietary intakes that are low in energy, protein, vitamin A, iron, riboflavin and calcium.

Rural family consuming a rice-based meal

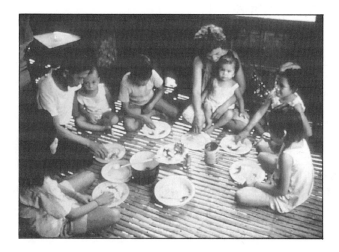

TABLE 10

Comparative daily provisional supply of nutrients per caput in developing and developed countries, 1986-88

Region	Energy (kcal)	Protein (g)	Fat (g)	Calcium (mg)	Iron (mg)	Vitamin A (µg retinol equivalents)	Thiamine (mg)	Riboflavin (mg)	Niacin (mg)	Ascorbic acid (mg)
World	2 671	70.0	65.8	472	14.4	900	1.39	1.01	15.4	94
Developed countries	3 398	102.7	128.7	860	16.1	1 329	1.61	1.68	20.9	138
Developing countries	2 434	59.4	45.4	346	13.9	760	1.31	0.79	13.5	80
Africa	2 119	51.1	37.4	363	17.8	859	1.37	0.80	13.8	89
Latin America	2 732	69.1	68.6	499	13.5	712	1.32	1.14	14.6	103
Near East	2 914	77.2	68.7	498	18.9	854	1.87	1.12	15.9	103
Far East	2 220	53.2	39.2	352	13.3	588	1.22	0.70	13.2	55
Others	2 379	51.3	61.8	402	14.3	1 342	1.16	1.06	15.4	202

Source: FAO, 1990b.

TABLE 11

Daily per caput nutrient supply in 36 countries with rice as staple

Country	Energy (*kcal*)	Protein (*g*)	Fat (*g*)	Calcium (*mg*)	Iron (*mg*)	Retinol (*μg*)	Thiamin (*mg*)	Riboflavin (*mg*)	Niacin (*mg*)	Ascorbic acid (*mg*)
Bangladesh	1 996	43.0	17.5	134	7.49	40	7.41	0.37	1.02	16
Belize	2 660	73.7	75.7	683	14.33	310	13.37	1.25	1.57	142
Brazil	2 722	60.4	76.0	479	11.23	330	10.17	1.02	1.18	134
Brunei	2 824	77.6	72.9	486	18.75	290	11.29	1.16	2.07	67
Cambodia	2 155	50.8	19.2	176	9.51	60	7.84	0.51	1.13	61
Colombia	2 571	57.0	60.6	487	14.59	290	11.00	1.10	1.48	96
Comoros	1 896	41.6	32.6	233	9.78	50	6.95	0.65	0.95	80
Côte d'Ivoire	2 580	54.4	54.0	333	13.28	120	13.90	0.80	1.75	201
Dominican Republic	2 342	47.1	61.9	382	10.03	160	8.48	0.94	1.25	88
Gambia	2 351	56.2	56.3	251	10.72	90	10.31	0.55	1.46	15
Guinea	2 192	51.2	45.8	262	11.86	60	11.57	0.65	1.29	247
Guinea-Bissau	2 471	50.8	55.2	189	9.94	80	9.55	0.64	1.27	43
Guyana	2 739	68.6	46.9	319	10.32	160	9.71	0.89	1.67	47
Hong Kong	2 817	85.4	109.1	389	15.04	420	12.99	1.12	1.73	83
India	2 197	53.2	38.9	417	14.93	70	14.27	0.79	1.41	55
Indonesia	2 709	59.7	39.1	226	11.94	50	10.15	0.53	1.40	58
Japan	2 909	94.2	78.9	610	15.86	480	13.38	1.21	1.67	114
Korea, DPR	2 798	80.3	36.6	352	16.43	80	15.70	0.99	1.82	136
Korea, Rep. of	2 853	76.8	59.0	501	16.88	160	14.04	0.97	1.59	168
Liberia	2 404	42.8	52.8	272	13.01	30	11.70	0.66	1.56	147
Madagascar	2 176	50.9	28.2	230	12.92	150	11.12	0.67	1.50	121
Malaysia	2 755	57.9	87.5	323	11.18	140	9.25	0.81	1.40	51
Maldives	2 375	89.2	39.7	387	17.64	60	11.95	1.09	2.80	72
Mauritius	2 823	67.3	58.0	505	13.06	250	10.59	1.02	1.29	29
Myanmar	2 474	63.9	40.4	219	10.27	60	8.70	0.51	1.16	39
Nepal	2 074	52.5	28.5	300	11.29	120	12.92	0.65	1.25	24

(continued)

TABLE 11 (continued)

Country	Energy (kcal)	Protein (g)	Fat (g)	Calcium (mg)	Iron (mg)	Retinol (µg)	Thiamin (mg)	Riboflavin (mg)	Niacin (mg)	Ascorbic acid (mg)
Papua New Guinea	2 410	48.8	41.4	403	14.56	90	13.37	1.26	1.64	309
Philippines	2 342	53.1	36.4	211	8.64	90	7.79	0.65	1.20	44
Seychelles	2 340	63.5	57.3	410	11.29	160	7.90	0.93	1.39	39
Sierra Leone	1 840	38.1	54.8	222	10.02	40	9.59	0.55	1.20	68
Singapore	3 248	91.1	78.5	533	15.62	280	16.89	1.28	2.09	92
Sri Lanka	2 298	46.3	43.0	334	12.45	50	7.11	0.58	0.96	67
Suriname	2 908	70.1	53.0	447	10.76	140	9.72	0.97	1.55	64
Thailand	2 312	49.0	39.0	198	9.23	90	8.22	0.56	1.15	56
Vanuatu	2 552	65.8	89.7	464	20.08	280	14.18	0.97	1.94	121
Viet Nam	2 232	50.5	28.2	170	8.62	70	7.65	0.54	1.09	74

Source: FAO Statistics Division, 1987-89 average.

General nutritional status

Table 13 provides information on some important indicators of overall nutritional status for 34 rice-consuming countries (UNICEF, 1991). It clearly indicates that in most of these countries the incidence of low birth weight, infant mortality and mortality under five is high and the prevalence of moderately and severely underweight children is alarmingly higher. The life expectancy is also low. About half the people in South Asia and sub-Saharan Africa receive inadequate energy for an active working life. Some 470 million undernourished people live in South Asia. All these data are a reflection of the poor general nutritional status of the population.

Protein-energy malnutrition

Protein-energy malnutrition still prevails widely in many rice-consuming countries. The low-income developing countries among the group are primarily and seriously affected. PEM is manifested by widespread growth retardation among preschool children. For example, nutrition surveys have

TABLE 12

Average daily energy and protein intake in selected rice-consuming countries

Country	Year of data collection	Energy intake (*kcal/caput/day*)	Protein intake (*g/caput/day*)
Bangladesh	1980/81	1 943	48.0
China	1982	2 485	67.0
Colombia	1981	2 223	55.3
Côte d'Ivoire	1979	2 140	55.7
Guyana	1976	2 054	55.5
Indonesia	1980	1 800	43.0
Madagascar	1962	2 223	55.3
Mauritius	1983	3 043	79.4
Nepal	1985	2 440	66.0
Philippines	1987	1 753	49.7
Sri Lanka	1980/81	2 030	49.9
Viet Nam	1988	2 142	59.1

Source: FAO country profiles and national nutrition surveys.

shown combined prevalence rates of 71 and 17 percent for moderate and severe underweight among preschool children in Bangladesh and the Philippines, respectively. In many other rice-consuming countries, particularly India, Laos, Madagascar, Nepal, Sierra Leone, Sri Lanka and Viet Nam, PEM is a major factor directly or indirectly contributing to high under-five mortality.

Vitamin A deficiency
Vitamin A deficiency is widespread in rice-consuming populations of tropical Asia (DeMaeyer, 1986). The most severely affected countries include Bangladesh, India, Indonesia, Myanmar, Nepal, the Philippines, Sri Lanka and Viet Nam. Vitamin A deficiency is also a problem in northeastern Brazil.

TABLE 13

Nutrition indicators for some selected rice-consuming countries

Country[a]	Under-five mortality[b] 1989	Infant mortality[c] 1989	Percent low birth-weight[d] 1980-88	Percent moderate and severe underweight, children 0-4 yr[e] 1980-89	Life expectancy[f] 1989	Daily per caput energy supply as percent of requirement 1984-86
Sierra Leone	261	151	17	21	42	81
Guinea	241	142	–	–	43	77
Bhutan	193	125	–	38	49	–
Bangladesh	184	116	28	71	51	83
Madagascar	179	117	10	33	54	106
Pakistan	162	106	25	52	57	95
Laos	156	106	39	37	49	104
India	145	96	30	41	59	100
Côte d'Ivoire	139	93	14	12	53	110
Indonesia	100	73	14	51	61	116
Guatemala	97	56	14	34	63	105
Myanmar	91	67	16	38	61	119
Brazil	85	61	8	5	65	111
Viet Nam	84	61	18	42	62	105
Dominican Republic	80	63	16	35	66	96
Philippines	72	44	18	33	64	104
Colombia	50	39	8	12	69	110
China	43	31	9	21	70	111
Korea, DPR	36	27	–	–	70	135
Sri Lanka	36	27	28	38	71	110
Thailand	35	21	12	26	66	105
Panama	33	23	8	16	72	107
Korea, Republic of	31	24	9	–	70	122
Malaysia	30	23	10	–	72	121

(continued)

TABLE 13 (continued)

Country[a]	Under-five mortality[b] 1989	Infant mortality[c] 1989	Percent low birth-weight[d] 1980-88	Percent moderate and severe underweight, children 0-4 yr[e] 1980-89	Life expectancy[f] 1989	Daily per caput energy supply as percent of requirement 1984-86
Mauritius	29	22	9	24	70	121
Singapore	12	8	7	14	74	124
Hong Kong	9	7	5	–	77	121
Japan	6	4	5	–	79	122

[a] Listed in descending order of under-five mortality rate.
[b] Annual number of deaths of children under five years of age per 1 000 live births.
[c] Annual number of deaths of children under one year of age per 1 000 live births.
[d] 2 500 g or less.
[e] Below minus two standard deviations from median weight for age of reference population.
[f] The number of years new-born children would live if subject to the mortality risks prevailing for the cross-section of population at the time of their birth.
Source: UNICEF, 1991.

Although it is difficult to determine the exact number of new cases of vitamin A deficiency and xerophthalmia occurring globally each year, available data from Indonesia indicated an annual rate of 2.7 per 1 000 children, leading to an estimate of 63 000 new cases annually for Indonesia. If a similar rate is applied to Bangladesh, India and the Philippines some 400 000 preschool children in these countries are likely to develop active corneal lesions resulting in total or partial blindness. It has been further estimated that worldwide some 3 million children under 10 years of age are currently suffering from blindness from xerophthalmia, about 1 million of whom are in India. In addition, countless children not presenting active signs of xerophthalmia are vitamin A depleted, a condition associated with decreased resistance to infectious diseases and increased mortality and morbidity.

Nutritional anaemias

Nutritional anaemias, mostly from iron deficiency, are widespread among rice-consuming countries. The causes are low dietary intake of iron, low biological availability of iron from food (Hallberg *et al.*, 1977), blood loss caused by intestinal parasites, particularly hookworm, and unfulfilled increased demand associated with rapid growth and pregnancy.

Anaemia is a condition diagnosed when haemoglobin level is below a set level suggested by the World Health Organization (WHO), depending on the age, sex and physiological condition (with adjustments necessary for high altitudes). A WHO estimate for 1980 (DeMaeyer and Adiels-Tegman, 1985) indicated that about 1 300 million of the 4 400 million people in the world suffer from anaemia and 1 200 million of these are from developing countries. Young children and pregnant women are most affected, with global prevalence rates estimated at 43 percent and 51 percent respectively, followed by school age children (37 percent), women of reproductive age (35 percent) and male adults (17 percent).

The highest overall prevalence of anaemia in the developing countries occurs in South Asia and Africa. The prevalence rate of anaemia in South Asia (DeMaeyer and Adiels-Tegman, 1985) was estimated to be 56 percent in children up to 4 years of age, 50 percent in 5- to 12-year-old children and 32 percent in men and 58 percent in women 15 to 59 years old. A higher rate (65 percent) was reported for pregnant women. Slightly lower rates were reported for East Asia, excluding China.

Estimates of anaemia from folate and vitamin B_{12} deficiency are not known, but this type of anaemia is reported to occur, particularly in India. Dietary patterns suggest increased risk in parts of Southeast Asia, but data are inadequate to confirm this.

Anaemia is an important cause of maternal mortality associated with childbirth. In addition, in adults it lowers work performance and has been linked with reduced immune competence and resistance to infection. Mild anaemia may also have far-reaching effects on psychological function and cognitive development.

Iodine deficiency disorders

Iodine deficiency disorder (IDD) is prevalent in many rice-eating populations, particularly in mountainous regions in Brazil, China, India, Indonesia and Malaysia, where the iodine content of soil, water and food is generally low

(Chong, 1979; Khor, Tee and Kandiah, 1990). IDD is also prevalent in Bangladesh because frequent flooding washes the iodine from the soil. It has been estimated that about 800 million people worldwide are at risk of IDD (United Nations, 1987). Nearly a quarter of those at risk have goitre and over 3 million are estimated to show overt cretinism. Most people at risk are in Asia, including 300 million in China and 200 million in India.

In areas with very high prevalence of iodine deficiency goitre may affect over 50 percent of the population and occurrence of cretinism may vary from 1 to 5 percent. An additional 25 percent may suffer from measurable impairment of mental and motor function. In some remote areas of the Himalayas IDD prevalence of 30 percent has been recorded.

Iodine is essential for normal growth and foetal development and for normal physical and mental activities in adults. Apart from overt signs of IDD, iodine-deficient populations may suffer from a variety of consequences that include reduced mental functions, widespread lethargy, increased stillbirths and increased infant mortality.

Thiamine and riboflavin deficiency

Thiamine and riboflavin deficiencies still exist in many parts of Asia. Beriberi is a characteristic disease of rice-eating communities, particularly when polished rice is consumed. It is rarely seen in communities where rice is eaten parboiled or undermilled. The replacement of hand pounding by machine mills in rural areas has aggravated the problem (Chong, 1979). Thiamine and riboflavin availabilities are lowest in Far Eastern diets (FAO, 1990b), (Table 10).

Clinical and experimental studies have suggested that the development of clinical manifestations of beriberi requires a thiamine intake below 0.2 mg per 1 000 kcal. Biochemical signs may be present at intakes as high as 0.3 mg per 1 000 kcal.

Over the years beriberi has tended to disappear as economic conditions have improved and diet has become more varied. Although the prevalence of clinical cases of apparent beriberi in adults has fallen, in many places beriberi in breast-fed infants is seen sporadically in some populations. For example, some rural lactating Thai mothers who only eat rice and salt postpartum and who restrict nutritious food are prone to develop thiamine deficiency. The low thiamine content in their breast milk predisposes their breast-fed infants to beriberi.

Angular stomatitis, a clinical sign often attributed to riboflavin deficiency, is also frequently seen in young children, pregnant women and lactating mothers in rice-eating populations in Bangladesh, India and Thailand. In Thai villages riboflavin deficiency has been reported to coexist with thiamine deficiency (Tanphaichitr, 1985).

Chapter 3
Grain structure, composition and consumers' criteria for quality

The rice grain (rough rice or paddy) consists of an outer protective covering, the hull, and the rice caryopsis or fruit (brown, cargo, dehulled or dehusked rice), (Juliano and Bechtel, 1985), (Figure 2). Brown rice consists of the outer layers of pericarp, seed-coat and nucellus; the germ or embryo; and the endosperm. The endosperm consists of the aleurone layer and the endosperm proper, consisting of the subaleurone layer and the starchy or inner endosperm. The aleurone layer encloses the embryo. Pigment is confined to the pericarp (Juliano and Bechtel, 1985).

The hull (husk) constitutes about 20 percent of the rough rice weight, but values range from 16 to 28 percent. The distribution of brown rice weight is pericarp 1 to 2 percent, aleurone plus nucellus and seed-coat 4 to 6 percent, germ 1 percent, scutellum 2 percent and endosperm 90 to 91 percent (Juliano, 1972).

The aleurone layer varies from one to five cell layers; it is thicker at the dorsal than at the ventral side and thicker in short-grain than in long-grain rices (del Rosario *et al.*, 1968). The aleurone and embryo cells are rich in protein bodies, containing globoids or phytate bodies, and in lipid bodies (Tanaka *et al.*, 1973; Tanaka, Ogawa and Kasai, 1977).

The endosperm cells are thin-walled and packed with amyloplasts containing compound starch granules. The two outermost cell layers (the subaleurone layer) are rich in protein and lipid and have smaller amyloplasts and compound starch granules than the inner endosperm. The starch granules are polyhedral and mainly 3 to 9 μm in size, with unimodal distribution. Protein occurs mainly in the form of spherical protein bodies 0.5 to 4 μm in size throughout the endosperm (del Rosario *et al.*, 1968;

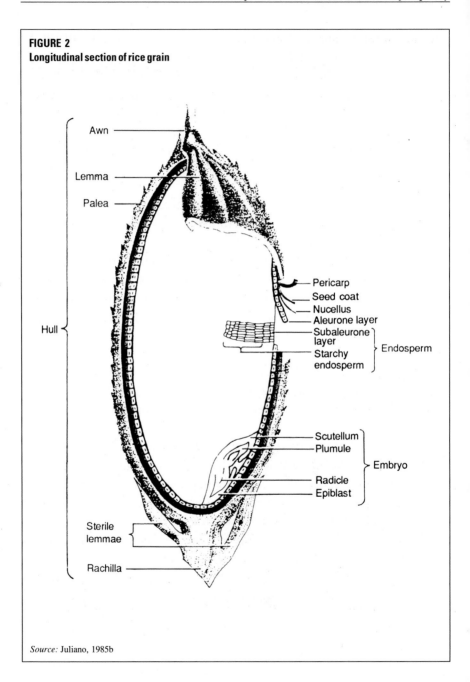

FIGURE 2
Longitudinal section of rice grain

Source: Juliano, 1985b

Bechtel and Pomeranz, 1978), (Figure 3), but crystalline protein bodies and small spherical protein bodies are localized in the subaleurone layer. The large spherical protein body corresponds to PB-I of Tanaka *et al.* (1980) and the crystalline protein body is identical to PB-II. Both PB-I and PB-II are distributed throughout the rice endosperm.

Non-waxy rice (containing amylose in addition to amylopectin) has a translucent endosperm, whereas waxy (0 to 2 percent amylose) rice has an opaque endosperm because of the presence of pores between and within the starch granules. Thus, waxy grain has about 95 to 98 percent the grain weight of non-waxy grain.

RICE CLASSIFICATION

There is no international standard for brown rice grain size and shape. IRRI uses the following scale for size: extra long, >7.50 mm; long, 6.61 to 7.50 mm; medium, 5.51 to 6.60 mm; and short, <5.50 mm. Grain shape is characterized based on length-to-width ratio: slender, >3.0; medium, 2.1 to 3.0; bold 1.1 to 2.0; and round, ≤1.0.

FIGURE 3
Schematic diagram of various protein bodies and compound starch granule in the endosperm subaleurone layer

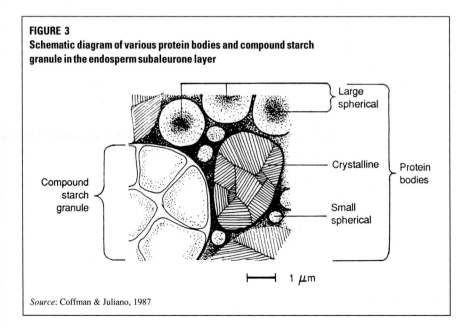

Source: Coffman & Juliano, 1987

The Codex Alimentarius Commission committee considering the draft standard for rice proposed the following classification of milled rice based on length-to-width ratio; long grain, ≤3.1; medium grain, 2.1 to 3.0; and short grain, ≤2.0 (Codex Alimentarius Commission, 1990).

Proposed tolerances for defects for milled rices are 0.5 percent each for organic and inorganic extraneous matter, 0.3 percent for rough rice, 1.0 percent each for brown rice and waxy rice, 2.0 percent for immature grains, 3.0 percent each for damaged and heat-damaged grains, 4.0 percent for red grains, 8.0 percent for red-streaked grains and 11.0 percent for chalky grains (Codex Alimentarius Commission, 1990). The proposed tolerances for milled parboiled rices are identical to those for milled rices except for no tolerance for chalky grains, 6.0 percent for heat-damaged grains and additional tolerances of 2.0 percent each for raw milled rice and pecks (grains with >25 percent of the surface coloured dark brown to black). A more detailed description of milling is given in Chapter 4.

GROSS NUTRIENT COMPOSITION

Among the milling fractions of rice, the bran has the highest energy and protein content and the hull has the lowest (Table 14). Only the brown rice fraction is edible. Abrasive or friction milling to remove the pericarp, seed-coat, testa, aleurone layer and embryo to yield milled rice results in loss of fat, protein, crude and neutral detergent fibre, ash, thiamine, riboflavin, niacin and α-tocopherol. Available carbohydrates, mainly starch, are higher in milled rice than in brown rice. The gradients for the various nutrients are not identical as evidenced from analysis of successive milling fractions of brown rice and milled rice (Barber, 1972), (Figure 4). Dietary fibre is highest in the bran layer (and the hull) and lowest in milled rice. Density and bulk density are lowest in the hull, followed by the bran, and highest in milled rice because of the low oil content. The nutritional properties of the rice grain are discussed further in Chapter 4.

The B vitamins are concentrated in the bran layers, as is α-tocopherol (vitamin E), (Table 15). The rice grain has no vitamin A, vitamin D or vitamin C (FAO, 1954). The locational gradient in the whole rice grain is steeper for thiamine than for riboflavin and niacin, resulting in a lower

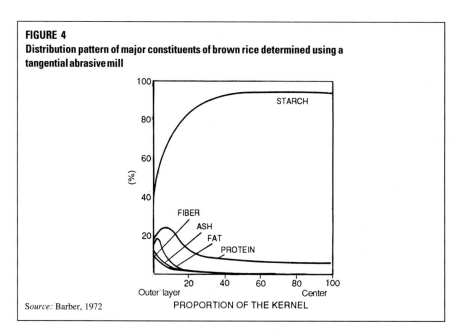

FIGURE 4
Distribution pattern of major constituents of brown rice determined using a tangential abrasive mill

Source: Barber, 1972

percent retention of thiamine (vitamin B_1) in milled rice (Table 15). About 50 percent of the total thiamine is in the scutellum and 80 to 85 percent of the niacin is in the pericarp plus aleurone layer (Hinton and Shaw, 1954). The embryo accounts for more than 95 percent of total tocopherols (of which α-tocopherols account for one-third) and nearly one-third of the oil content of the rice grain (Gopala Krishna, Prabhakar and Sen, 1984). By calculation, 65 percent of the thiamine of brown rice is in the bran, 13 percent in the polish and 22 percent in the milled rice fraction (Juliano and Bechtel, 1985). Corresponding values for riboflavin are 39 percent in the bran, 8 percent in the polish and 53 percent in the milled rice fraction. Niacin distribution is 54 percent in the bran, 13 percent in the polish and 33 percent in the milled rice fraction.

The minerals (ash) are also concentrated in the outer layers of brown rice or in the bran fraction (Table 15). A major proportion (90 percent) of the phosphorus in bran is phytin phosphorus. Potassium and magnesium are the principal salts of phytin. The ash distribution in brown rice is 51 percent in the bran, 10 percent in the germ, 10 percent in the polish and 28 percent in

TABLE 14
Proximate composition of rough rice and its milling fractions at 14 percent moisture

Rice fraction	Crude protein (g N x 5.95)	Crude fat (g)	Crude fibre (g)	Crude ash (g)	Available carbo- hydrates (g)	Neutral detergent fibre (g)	Energy content		Density (g/ml)	Bulk density (g/ml)
							(kJ)	(kcal)		
Rough rice	5.8-7.7	1.5-2.3	7.2-10.4	2.9-5.2	64-73	16.4-19.2	1 580	378	1.17-1.23	0.56-0.64
Brown rice	7.1-8.3	1.6-2.8	0.6-1.0	1.0-1.5	73-87	2.9-3.9	1 520-1 610	363-385	1.31	0.68
Milled rice	6.3-7.1	0.3-0.5	0.2-0.5	0.3-0.8	77-89	0.7-2.3	1 460-1 560	349-373	1.44-1.46	0.78-0.85
Rice bran	11.3-14.9	15.0-19.7	7.0-11.4	6.6-9.9	34-62	24-29	670-1 990	399-476	1.16-1.29	0.20-0.40
Rice hull	2.0-2.8	0.3-0.8	34.5-45.9	13.2-21.0	22-34	66-74	1 110-1 390	265-332	0.67-0.74	0.10-0.16

Sources: Juliano, 1985b; Eggum, Juliano & Maniñgat, 1982; Pedersen & Eggum, 1983.

TABLE 15
Vitamin and mineral content of rough rice and its milling fractions at 14 percent moisture

Rice fraction	Thiamine (mg)	Riboflavin (mg)	Niacin (mg)	α-Tocopherol (mg)	Calcium (mg)	Phosphorus (g)	Phytin P (g)	Iron (mg)	Zinc (mg)
Rough rice	0.26-0.33	0.06-0.11	2.9-5.6	0.90-2.00	10-80	0.17-0.39	0.18-0.21	1.4-6.0	1.7-3.1
Brown rice	0.29-0.61	0.04-0.14	3.5-5.3	0.90-2.50	10-50	0.17-0.43	0.13-0.27	0.2-5.2	0.6-2.8
Milled rice	0.02-0.11	0.02-0.06	1.3-2.4	75-0.30	10-30	0.08-0.15	0.02-0.07	0.2-2.8	0.6-2.3
Rice bran	1.20-2.40	0.18-0.43	26.7-49.9	2.60-13.3	30-120	1.1-2.5	0.9-2.2	8.6-43.0	4.3-25.8
Rice hull	0.09-0.21	0.05-0.07	1.6-4.2	0	60-130	0.03-0.07	0	3.9-9.5	0.9-4.0

Sources: Juliano, 1985; Pedersen & Eggum, 1983.

TABLE 16

Amino acid content of rough rice and its milling fractions at 14 percent moisture (g per 16 g N)

Rice fraction	Histidine	Isoleucine	Leucine	Lysine	Methionine + cysteine	Phenylalanine + tyrosine	Threonine	Tryptophan	Valine	Amino acid score[a] (%)
Rough rice	1.5-2.8	3.0-4.8	6.9-8.8	3.2-4.7	4.5-6.2	9.3-10.8	3.0-4.5	1.2-2.0	4.6-7.0	55-81
Brown rice	2.3-2.5	3.4-4.4	7.9-8.5	3.7-4.1	4.4-4.6	8.6-9.3	3.7-3.8	1.2-1.4	4.8-6.3	64-71
Milled rice	2.2-2.6	3.5-4.6	8.0-8.2	3.2-4.0	4.3-5.0	9.3-10.4	3.5-3.7	1.2-1.7	4.7-6.5	55-69
Rice bran	2.7-3.3	2.7-4.1	6.9-7.6	4.8-5.4	4.2-4.8	7.7-8.0	3.8-4.2	0.6-1.2	4.9-6.0	83-93
Rice hull	1.6-2.0	3.2-4.0	8.0-8.2	3.8-5.4	3.5-3.7	6.6-7.3	4.2-5.0	0.6	5.5-7.5	66-93

[a] Based on 5.8 g lysine per 16 g N as 100% (WHO, 1985).
Sources: Juliano, 1985b; Eggum, Juliano & Maniñgat, 1982; Pedersen & Eggum, 1983.

the milled rice fraction; iron, phosphorus and potassium show a similar distribution (Resurrección, Juliano and Tanaka, 1979). However, some minerals show a relatively more even distribution in the grain: milled rice retained 63 percent of the sodium, 74 percent of the calcium and 83 percent of the Kjeldahl N content of brown rice (Juliano, 1985b).

The amino acid content of the milling fractions is given in Table 16.

Starch

Starch is the major constituent of milled rice at about 90 percent of the dry matter. Starch is a polymer of D-glucose linked α-(1-4) and usually consists of an essentially linear fraction, amylose, and a branched fraction, amylopectin. Branch points are α-(1-6) linkages. Innovative techniques have now shown rice amylose to have two to four chains with a number-average degree of polymerization $(\overline{DP}_n)$ of 900 to 1 100 glucose units and a ß-amylolysis limit of 73 to 87 percent (Hizukuri *et al.*, 1989). It is a mixture of branched and linear molecules with $\overline{DP}_n$ of 1 100 to 1 700 and 700 to 900, respectively. The branched fraction constitutes 25 to 50 percent by number and 30 to 60 percent by weight of amylose. The iodine affinity of rice amyloses is 20 to 21 percent by weight.

Rice amylopectins have ß-amylolysis limits of 56 to 59 percent, chain lengths of 19 to 22 glucose units, $\overline{DP}_n$ of 5 000 to 15 000 glucose units and 220 to 700 chains per molecule (Hizukuri *et al.*, 1989). The iodine affinity of rice amylopectin is 0.4 to 0.9 percent in low- and intermediate-amylose rices but 2 to 3 percent in high-amylose rices. Isoamylase-debranched amylopectins showed more longest chain fractions $(\overline{DP}_n > 100)$ (9 to 14 percent) in high-amylose samples with higher iodine affinity than in low- and intermediate-amylose samples (2 to 5 percent) and waxy rice amylopectin (0 percent), (Hizukuri *et al.*, 1989).

Based on colorimetric starch-iodine colour absorption standards at 590 to 620 nm, milled rice is classified as waxy (1 to 2 percent), very low amylose (2 to 12 percent), low amylose (12 to 20 percent), intermediate (20 to 25 percent) and high (25 to 33 percent), (Juliano, 1979, 1985b). Recent collaborative studies showed that the maximum true amylose content is 20 percent and that additional iodine binding is due to the long linear chains in amylopectin (Takeda, Hizukuri and Juliano, 1987). Hence colorimetric amylose values are now termed "apparent amylose content".

The waxy endosperm is opaque and shows air spaces between the starch granules, which have a lower density than non-waxy granules. The structure of the starch granule is still not well understood, but crystallinity and staling are attributed to the amylopectin fraction.

Protein

Protein is determined by first carrying out micro Kjeldahl digestion and ammonia distillation and then using titration or colorimetric ammonia assay of the digest to determine nitrogen content, which is converted to protein by the factor 5.95. [The factor, based on a nitrogen content of 16.8 percent for the major protein of milled rice (glutelin), may be an overestimation; reappraisals have suggested values of 5.1 to 5.5 (5.17 ± 0.25) (Mossé, Huet and Baudet, 1988; Mossé, 1990), 5.24 to 5.66 (mean 5.37) (Hegsted and Juliano, 1974) and 5.61 (Sosulski and Imafidon, 1990).]

Endosperm (milled rice) protein consists of several fractions comprising 15 percent albumin (water soluble) plus globulin (salt soluble), 5 to 8 percent prolamin (alcohol soluble) and the rest glutelin (alkali soluble), (Juliano, 1985b). Using sequential protein extraction, the mean ratio for 33 samples was found to be 9 percent prolamin, 7 percent albumin plus globulin and 84 percent glutelin (Huebner *et al.*, 1990). The mean prolamin content of seven IRRI milled rices was 6.5 percent of their total protein (IRRI, 1991b). The lysine content of rice protein is 3.5 to 4.0 percent, one of the highest among cereal proteins.

Rice bran proteins are richer in albumin than endosperm proteins and are found as distinct protein bodies containing globoids in the aleurone layer and the germ. These structures are different from endosperm protein bodies. Tanaka *et al.* (1973) reported the presence of 66 percent albumin, 7 percent globulin and 27 percent prolamin plus glutelin in aleurone protein bodies. Ogawa, Tanaka and Kasai (1977) reported the presence of 98 percent albumin in embryo protein bodies.

The endosperm protein is localized mainly in protein bodies (Figure 4). The crystalline (PB-II) protein bodies are rich in glutelin, and the large spherical protein bodies (PB-I) are rich in prolamin. Ogawa *et al.* (1987) estimated that endosperm storage proteins were composed of 60 to 65 percent PB-II proteins, 20 to 25 percent PB-I proteins and 10 to 15 percent albumin and globulin in the cytoplasm.

Rice starch granule amylose binds up to 0.7 percent protein that is mainly the waxy gene protein or granule-bound starchy synthase, with a molecular mass of about 60 kilodaltons (kd), (Villareal and Juliano, 1989b).

Rice glutelin consists of three acidic or α subunits of 30 to 39 kd and two basic or ß subunits of 19 to 25 kd (Kagawa, Hirano and Kikuchi, 1988). The two kinds of subunits are formed by cleavage of a 57-kd polypeptide precursor (Sugimoto, Tanaka and Kasai, 1986). Prolamin consists mainly (90 percent) of the 13-kd subunit plus two minor subunits of 10 and 16 kd (Hibino *et al.*, 1989).

The essential amino acid contents of the glutelin and prolamin subunits (Table 17) showed lysine as limiting in these polypeptides except in the IEF3 fraction of the 13-kd prolamin subunit, which has 5.5 percent lysine and is limiting in methionine plus cysteine. Thus, glutelin has a better amino acid score than prolamin except for the 16-kd prolamin subunit. The 10-kd prolamin subunit has a high (6.8 percent) cysteine content.

Lipid

The lipid or fat content of rice is mainly in the bran fraction (20 percent, dry basis), specifically as lipid bodies or spherosomes in the aleurone layer and bran; however, about 1.5 to 1.7 percent is present in milled rice, mainly as non-starch lipids extracted by ether, chloroform-methanol and cold water-saturated butanol (Juliano and Goddard, 1986; Tanaka *et al.*, 1978). Protein bodies, particularly the core, are rich in lipids (Choudhury and Juliano, 1980; Tanaka *et al.*, 1978). The major fatty acids of these lipids are linoleic, oleic and palmitic acids (Hemavathy and Prabhaker, 1987; Taira, Nakagahra and Nagamine, 1988). Essential fatty acids in rice oil are about 29 to 42 percent linoleic acid and 0.8 to 1.0 percent linolenic acid (Jaiswal, 1983). The content of essential fatty acids may be increased with temperature during grain development, but at the expense of reduction in total oil content (Taira, Taira and Fujii, 1979).

TABLE 17

Aminogram (g/16 g N) of the acidic and basic subunits of rice glutelin and the major and minor subunits of prolamin

Amino acid	Glutelin subunits[a]		Prolamin subunits		
	30-39 kd (acidic)	19-25 kd (basic)	13 kd	10 kd	16 kd
Histidine	2.2-2.5	2.6-2.7	2.0-2.4	1.7	4.2
Isoleucine	3.2-3.3	4.1-4.9	3.8-5.4	1.6	3.6
Leucine	6.4-7.5	7.0-8.5	17.9-26.4	4.7	8.1
Lysine	2.2-3.0	3.0-4.1	0.4-5.5	1.0	3.3
Methionine + cystine[b]	0.2-1.9	0.1-2.4	0.7-1.2	22.5	5.3
Phenylalanine + tyrosine	10.0-10.5	10.1-10.8	12.7-21.6	4.3	7.6
Threonine	2.8-3.7	2.5-3.7	1.8-2.8	6.8	2.7
Valine	5.1-5.7	5.7-7.0	2.7-3.9	4.4	3.9
Amino acid score[c] (%)	38-52	52-71	7-8[d]	18	57

[a] S-cyanoethyl glutelin subunits.
[b] Only the IEF3 fraction of the 13-kd, 10-kd and 16-kd prolamin subunits had cystine. All glutelins had substituted cysteine residues.
[c] Based on 5.8% lysine as 100% (WHO, 1985).
[d] Alternative value is 34% based on 2.5% methionine + cysteine as 100% (WHO, 1985).
Sources: Juliano & Boulter, 1976; Villareal & Juliano, 1978 (glutelin subunits); Hibino *et al.*, 1989 (prolamin subunits).

Starch lipids are mainly monoacyl lipids (fatty acids and lysophosphatides) complexed with amylose (Choudhury and Juliano, 1980). The starch lipid content is lowest for waxy starch granules (≤ 0.2 percent). It is highest for intermediate-amylose rices (1.0 percent) and may be slightly lower in high-amylose rice (Choudhury and Juliano, 1980; Juliano and Goddard, 1986). Waxy milled rice has more non-starch lipids than non-waxy rice. Starch lipids are protected from oxidative rancidity, and the amylose-lipid complex is digested by growing rats (Holm *et al.*, 1983). However, starch lipids contribute little to the energy content of the rice grain. The major fatty acids of starch lipids are palmitic and linoleic acids, with lesser amounts of oleic acid (Choudhury and Juliano, 1980).

TABLE 18

Yield and composition of defatted and protease-amylase treated cell wall preparations obtained from different histological fractions of milling of brown rice

Rice fraction	Yield (% defatted tissue)	Composition (% of total)				Uronic acid in pectin (%)	Arabinose:xylose ratio	
		Pectic substances	Hemi-cellulose	α–cellulose	Lignin		Pectic substances	Hemi-cellulose
Caryopsis coat	29	7	38	27	32	32	1.63	0.82
Aleurone tissue	20	11	42	16	25	25	1.78	0.84
Germ	12	23	47	9	16	16	2.29	0.96
Endosperm	0.3	27	49	1	34	34	1.09	0.64

Source: Shibuya, 1989.

Non-starch polysaccharides

Non-starch polysaccharides consist of water soluble polysaccharides and insoluble dietary fibre (Juliano, 1985b). They can complex with starch and may have a hypocholesterolaemic effect (Normand, Ory and Mod, 1981; Normand *et al.*, 1984). The endosperm has a lower content of dietary fibre than the rest of brown rice (Shibuya, 1989), (Table 18). Reported values for neutral detergent fibre are 0.7 to 2.3 percent (Juliano, 1985b), (Table 14). In addition, the endosperm or milled rice cell wall has a low lignin content but a high content of pectic substances or pectin. Endosperm pectin has a higher uronic acid content but a lower arabinose-to-xylose ratio than the other grain tissues. The hemicellulose of endosperm also has a lower arabinose-to-xylose ratio than the three other grain tissues.

Volatiles

The volatiles characteristic of cooked rice are ammonia, hydrogen sulphide and acetaldehyde (Obata and Tanaka, 1965). Upon cooking, all aromatic rices contain 2-acetyl-1-pyrroline as the major aromatic principle (Buttery *et al.*, 1983). Volatiles characteristic of fat rancidity are aldehydes, particularly hexanal, and ketones.

ENVIRONMENTAL INFLUENCE ON RICE COMPOSITION

Environmental factors are known to affect the composition of the rice grain (Juliano, 1985b). Protein content tends to increase with wider spacing or in borders and in response to high N fertilizer application, especially at flowering. Short growth duration and cloudy weather during grain development, as occurs in the wet season, may increase protein content. Stresses such as drought, salinity, alkalinity, high or low temperature, diseases or pests may increase the protein content of the rice grain. An increase in protein content is essentially at the expense of a reduction in starch content.

Environmental factors that increase protein content, such as soil type, ambient temperature during ripening and growth duration, also increase the ash content of brown rice but have no effect on its fat content. Mineral nutrition affects the protein content of the rice grain: soil organic matter, total nitrogen, exchangeable calcium, available copper and molybdenum and total chlorine all tend to increase the grain protein content (Huang, 1990).

As growth duration increases, brown rice protein content decreases (IRRI, 1988b). By contrast, yield and brown rice protein were not always significantly negatively correlated.

Upland culture had a variable effect on the protein content of eight varieties of rice grown in Côte d'Ivoire; five showed a lower milled rice protein content and two showed a higher protein content under upland culture (Villareal, Juliano and Sauphanor, 1990).

In Punjab, Pakistan, high soil salinity increased the brown rice protein content in three of four varieties differing in salinity tolerance but had no effect on the protein content of the fourth (Siscar-Lee *et al.*, 1990). Soil sulphur deficiency reduces grain yield without having any adverse effect on the cysteine and methionine contents of the rice protein (Juliano *et al.*, 1987).

The mineral content of the grain is affected by the mineral content of the soil and of the irrigation water. For instance, pollution of irrigation water with mine tailings has resulted in high cadmium content in some Japanese rices which has proved to be harmful (Kitagishi and Yamane, 1981).

GRAIN QUALITY

Consumers' criteria

When more rice becomes available in the market, consumers' demand for superior quality rice is increased. Although sensory evaluations by laboratory panels and consumer panels give some indication on important criteria for rice quality, they do not reflect the properties for which consumers will actually pay a price premium in the retail market. By clearly identifying the quality characteristics valued by consumers, plant breeders can target attributes that are economically significant in breeding improvement research. The results could provide social scientists with an agenda for public policy research in rice marketing, technology assessment and research prioritization.

Rice grain quality denotes different properties to various groups in the post-harvest system (Juliano and Duff, 1989). Although variety is the principal factor contributing to grain quality, good post-harvest handling can maintain or even improve it (Table 19). Moisture content is the most important quality criterion for rough rice. To the farmer, grain quality refers to quality of seed for planting material and dry grain for consumption, with minimum moisture, microbial deterioration and spoilage. The miller or trader looks for low moisture, variety integrity and high total and head milled rice yield. Market quality is mainly determined by physical properties and variety name, whereas cooking and eating quality is determined by physico-chemical properties, particularly apparent amylose content. In countries with marked variability in temperatures during the ripening periods, significant differences in grain quality have been reported within a variety. In tropical Asia, grain physico-chemical properties are relatively constant. Nutritional value is mainly determined by the milled rice protein content.

The major findings of research on the economics of grain quality from 1987 to 1989 by IRRI and national rice research programmes in Indonesia, Bangladesh, Malaysia, the Philippines and Thailand are that rice grain quality and quality preferences vary across countries and regions but some quality preferences are widely shared (IRRI and IDRC, 1992). Consumers in all the countries studied prefer higher head rice yield and more translucent grain. High-income consumers pay higher premiums for a larger number of

TABLE 19

Effects of environment, processing and variety on rice grain properties influencing quality at different steps of the post-harvest system

Post-harvest process and associated grain property	Environment	Processing method	Variety
Harvesting	+[a]	+	+ (Growth duration, photoperiod, degree of ripening, dormancy)
Threshing	+	+	+ (Threshability, shattering)
Drying	+	+	+ (Crack resistance)
Yellowing	+	+	0
Storage/ageing	+	+	+ (Waxy rice ages less than non-waxy)
Parboiling	+	+	+ (Gelatinization temperature)
Pecky grain	+	+	+ (Stink-bug resistance)
Dehulling	0	+	+ (Hull tightness and content)
Milling			
Head rice	+	+	+ (Crack resistance)
Marketing			
Size and shape	+	0	+ (Genetically determined)
Degree of milling (whiteness)	+	+	+ (Depth of grooves)
Head rice	+	+	+ (Crack resistance)
Translucency	+	+	+
Aroma	+	+	+
Foreign matter	+	+	0
Shelf life	+	+	0
Cooking and eating			
Amylose content	+	0	+ (Volume expansion and texture)
Gelatinization temperature	+	0	+ (Cooking time)
Gel consistency	+	0	+
Texture of cooked rice	+	+	+
Grain elongation	+	+	+

[a]+, quality affected; 0, no effect.
Source: Juliano & Duff, 1989.

quality characteristics than low-income consumers, reflecting their ability to pay. Preferences do not vary much across income levels, with one exception: lower-income consumers prefer rice that is more filling. Laboratory analysis showed that Philippine rice labelled with a traditional variety name is usually a modern variety with shape or cooking characteristics similar to those of traditional varieties (Juliano *et al.*, 1989b). Thus, the "traditional" label signals consumers that these rices have some desirable characteristics.

Quality incentives appear to be transmitted from wholesale rice prices through to rough rice prices in Indonesia and the Philippines (IRRI and IDRC, 1992). However, this transmission is not perfect. The Philippine studies show that barriers to entry in milling influence pricing efficiency. The studies reveal the complexity of the transmission of information about quality from consumers to producers.

Given the importance of quality characteristics for creating and stimulating demand, especially among the higher-income urban sector, transmission of price and market signals and a greater degree of integration of the farm wholesale and retail market will be necessary to improve the farmgate price and to provide incentive to farmers to produce better-quality rice. Moreover, improvements in grain quality that do not lower yields will generally benefit all rice consumers by lowering the cost of better-quality rice (Unnevehr *et al.*, 1985). If higher-quality varieties are widely adopted, producers will benefit by retaining better-quality rice for home consumption and by having a wider domestic market for their products. In addition, countries exporting rice would benefit from quality improvements that would expand their potential export market.

Grain quality indicators

Physical properties such as length, width, translucency, degree of milling, colour and age of milled rice are grain quality indicators. The amylose content of the rice starch is the major eating quality factor. It correlates directly with volume expansion and water absorption during cooking and with hardness, whiteness and dullness of cooked rice (Juliano, 1985b). Genetic studies showed that the non-waxy trait is dominant over the waxy trait (Kumar, Khush and Juliano, 1987). Among non-waxy parents, high amylose is completely dominant over low or intermediate amylose, and intermediate is dominant over low (Kumar and Khush, 1987).

Final gelatinization temperature (GT) of starch granules refers to the water temperature at which at least 90 percent of the starch granules have gelatinized or lost birefringence (Maltese cross) or swollen irreversibly in hot water. GT is classified for rice starch granules as low (55 to 69.5°C), intermediate (70 to 74°C) and high (74.5 to 80°C). GT is indexed in the breeding programme by the alkali spreading value based on the degree of dispersion of six grains of milled rice in 10 ml of 1.7 percent potassium hydroxide after 23 hours soaking at 30°C (Little, Hilder and Dawson, 1958).

A high GT value is uncommon, particularly in high amylose rices. A low ambient temperature during ripening may increase amylose content and independently reduce GT (Nikuni *et al.*, 1969; Resurrección *et al.*, 1977; Dien *et al.*, 1987). The GT affects the degree of cooking of rice because of the cooking gradient from the surface to the core of the grain. Because GT correlates directly with cooking time, a low GT favours fuel conservation, provided eating quality is not adversely affected. GT also affects the molecular properties of amylopectin.

The gel consistency test was developed to index cooked rice hardness among high-amylose rices (Cagampang, Perez and Juliano, 1973). Rices are classified based on gel length as soft (61 to 100 mm), medium (41 to 60 mm) and hard (27 to 40 mm), (Table 18). Soft to medium gel consistency is preferred to hard gel consistency in both non-waxy and waxy rices. High protein content contributes to harder gel consistency. Amylopectin contributes more than amylose to starch gel consistency and viscosity.

Among rices of the same apparent amylose type, alkali spreading value and gel consistency may be used as quality indices. Among high-amylose rices, intermediate GT and soft gel consistency are preferred by consumers over low GT and hard gel consistency (Juliano, 1985b). Among intermediate-amylose rices derived from C4-63G, those with an intermediate GT value are preferred to those with a low GT value, as the cooked rice is softer. Gel consistency values are similar among these intermediate-amylose rices. Among low-amylose and waxy rices, a low-GT type is preferred to a type with a high GT value. In terms of rice improvement breeding, hard gel

TABLE 20
Relative importance of rice quality indicators in rice breeding programmes

Breeding programme	Physical properties[a]	Starch texture[b]	Cooked rice texture[b]
Traditional varieties	Main	Optional	Optional
Modern varieties	Major	Major	Verification
Grain quality	Major	Verification	Major

[a]Amylose content, alkali spreading value (gelatinization temperature), gel consistency.
[b]Determined by sensory evaluation or instrument — Instron, Texturometer, Tensipresser, Viscoelastograph, etc.
Source: Juliano & Duff, 1991.

consistency is dominant over medium and soft gel, and medium gel consistency is dominant over soft (Tang, Khush and Juliano, 1989).

As many countries achieve rice self-sufficiency, grain quality becomes an important breeding objective (Juliano and Duff, 1991). In traditional breeding programmes, both parents are of known quality so that the quality of the breeding lines is predictable by indicators based on physical properties, namely apparent amylose content, alkali spreading value and gel consistency (Table 20). With modern or semi-dwarf varieties, derived from parents of contrasting grain qualities, evaluation of starch properties complements physical methods in indexing quality of breeding lines. Breeding for grain quality involves discrimination among lines with similar starch properties, as in the United States, Japan and the Republic of Korea and at IRRI, where cooked rice texture is the key indicator.

Heritability of protein content is very low. A six-percentage-point range is observed for each variety (Coffman and Juliano, 1987). Environmental factors contribute significantly to protein content. High-protein rice trans-locates straw N to the developing grain more efficiently, which results in a higher N harvest index (panicle N/panicle N + straw N), (Perez *et al.*, 1973).

Quality characteristics of world rices - country samples
In Asian countries high-amylose rices predominate (Table 21). This is the principal rice type in Bangladesh, Sri Lanka, Thailand and Viet Nam.

TABLE 21

Amylose scattergram and protein content of milled rices of varieties grown in various countries in Asia (IRRI 1963-90)

Country	Number of samples	Waxy	Very low	Low	Inter-mediate	High	Range	Mean
		Amylose type[a]					Percent protein[b]	
Bangladesh	58	0	0	2	7	49	5-12	7.7
Bhutan	40	0	0	2	22	16	5-9	6.9
Brunei	11	0	1	0	4	6	6-13	7.9
Cambodia	34	0	0	4	5	25	4-12	6.4
China	74	4	0	18	12	40	6-13	8.3
Taiwan	58	10	0	34	6	8	4-11	7.6
India	52	0	0	2	8	42	6-11	8.5
Maharashtra	14	0	0	0	2	12	5-8	6.3
Indonesia	133	5	2	5	50	71	5-11	7.9
Iran	33	0	0	11	15	7	3-12	9.2
Japan	67	5	0	57	5	0	5-12	7.2
Korea, South	147	4	2	121	19	1	6-11	8.2
Laos	20	11	2	1	5	1	6-9	7.4
Malaysia								
Sarawak	27	0	3	4	6	14	5-14	7.1
Sabah	10	0	0	0	3	7	6-8	6.8
West Malaysia	46	3	0	0	5	38	6-11	7.4
Myanmar	61	1	11	12	19	18	5-11	6.9
Nepal	46	0	0	10	8	28	5-9	7.0
Pakistan	66	0	0	3	33	30	6-10	8.1
Philippines[c]	328	39	3	23	98	165	5-14	8.2
Sri Lanka	67	0	0	0	6	61	6-13	8.8
Thailand	83	22	2	6	13	40	4-14	8.0
Turkey	14	0	0	13	1	0	6-10	7.4
Viet Nam	133	1	0	6	24	102	5-11	7.7
Total	**1 622**	**105**	**26**	**334**	**376**	**781**	**4-14**	**7.8**

[a] Percent amylose, milled rice dry weight basis: waxy 0-5%, very low 5.1-12.0%, low 12.1-20.0%, intermediate 20.1-25.0%, high >25.0%.
[b] At 12% H_2O.
[c] Includes varieties grown at IRRI.
Source: Juliano & Villareal, 1991.

Intermediate-amylose rices predominate in Bhutan, Myanmar and Pakistan, whereas low-amylose rices predominate in Taiwan Province (China), Japan and the Republic of Korea. Very low amylose rices are identified only in Brunei, Indonesia, the Republic of Korea, Laos, Sarawak (Malaysia), Myanmar, the Philippines and Thailand. Waxy rices are represented in China, Indonesia, Japan, the Republic of Korea, Laos, West Malaysia, Myanmar, the Philippines and Thailand. Waxy rice is the staple in Laos and north and northeast Thailand.

Protein content in these milled rice samples ranged from 4 to 14 percent and mean protein ranged from 6.3 to 9.2 percent (Table 21). The overall mean protein content is 7.8 percent.

Of the varieties grown outside Asia, low-, intermediate- and high-amylose rices are equally represented (Table 22). High-amylose rices predominate in Colombia, Ghana, Guatemala, Nigeria, Paraguay, Peru, Sierra Leone and Venezuela. Intermediate-amylose rices predominate in Chile, Greece, Hungary, the Islamic Republic of Iran, Italy, Suriname and Venezuela. Low-amylose rices predominate in Argentina, Australia, Bulgaria, Egypt, France, Portugal, Turkey, the United States and the area of the former Soviet Union. The United States has the only very low amylose rice and has waxy rices as does Australia.

The protein content of milled rice samples grown outside Asia ranged from 5 to 13 percent and mean values ranged from 6.2 to 10.5 percent (Table 22). Mean protein is 7.2 percent, which is lower than that of Asian rice (Table 21).

The amylose types preferred in various rice-producing countries in Asia and elsewhere producing 0.1 percent or more of total world production are tabulated in Table 23 (Juliano and Duff, 1991). Intermediate-amylose rice seems the most popular, followed by low- and high-amylose rices and lastly waxy rice. Low-amylose rices were mainly japonica except in Thailand and Argentina. The Thai rices are the jasmine or Khao Dawk Mali 105 type that is becoming popular in the United States and Europe. Intermediate-amylose rices were preferred in the most countries; these include Basmati rices, Indonesian bulu (Javanica) varieties, Myanmar's Nga Kywe or D25-4 elongating rices and United States long-grain varieties. High-amylose rices

TABLE 22

Amylose scattergram and protein content of milled rices of varieties grown in various countries outside Asia (IRRI, 1963-90)

Country	Number of samples	Amylose type[a]					Percent protein[b]	
		Waxy	Very low	Low	Inter-mediate	High	Range	Mean
Argentina	46	0	0	23	16	7	6-9	7.6
Australia	25	2	0	13	7	3	5-10	6.7
Bolivia	6	0	0	1	5	0	7-10	8.2
Brazil	91	0	0	23	26	42	5-13	8.5
Bulgaria	23	0	0	14	8	1	6-10	7.4
Cameroon	2	0	0	0	1	1	8-11	9.8
Chile	14	0	0	5	4	0	6-10	7.4
Colombia	20	0	0	0	5	15	6-11	7.9
Costa Rica	4	0	0	0	2	2	9-13	10.5
Côte d'Ivoire	23	0	0	6	8	9	6-11	7.9
Cuba	24	0	0	7	7	10	6-9	7.6
Dominican Republic	9	0	0	1	2	6	4-9	7.6
Ecuador	17	0	0	0	3	14	6-8	6.8
Egypt	44	0	0	29	8	7	5-10	6.7
El Salvador	12	0	0	0	5	7	6-11	8.2
France	43	0	0	27	14	2	5-12	7.0
Ghana	22	0	0	0	7	15	6-9	7.8
Greece	10	0	0	3	5	2	5-8	6.4
Guatemala	8	0	0	0	2	6	6-8	6.8
Guyana	10	0	0	0	4	6	7-12	8.8
Hungary	42	0	0	15	26	1	6-11	7.2
Italy	37	0	0	14	23	0	5-8	6.9
Liberia	12	0	0	2	3	7	6-9	7.6
Madagascar	9	0	0	1	3	5	5-10	7.5
Mexico	35	0	0	1	12	22	5-11	7.2

(continued)

TABLE 22 (continued)

Country	Number of samples	Amylose type[a]					Percent protein[b]	
		Waxy	Very low	Low	Inter-mediate	High	Range	Mean
Nigeria	66	0	0	7	16	43	6-11	7.4
Panama	2	0	0	0	0	2	6	6.2
Paraguay	15	0	0	1	2	12	7-10	8.4
Peru	35	0	0	11	8	16	5-11	7.5
Portugal	31	0	0	17	13	1	5-8	6.8
Senegal	11	0	0	0	1	10	5-10	7.2
Sierra Leone	108	0	0	9	14	85	5-10	7.0
Soviet Union	25	0	0	16	9	0	5-7	6.4
Spain	12	0	0	9	3	0	6-13	8.2
Suriname	34	0	0	8	15	11	6-9	7.5
Togo	2	0	0	0	1	1	8	7.6
United States	87	5	1	40	23	18	5-10	7.0
Venezuela	6	0	0	0	0	6	6-7	7.1
Total	**1 017**	**7**	**1**	**303**	**316**	**390**	**5-13**	**7.2**

[a]Percent amylose, milled rice dry weight basis: waxy 0-5%, very low 5.1-12.0%, low 12.1-20.0%, intermediate 20.1-25.0%, high >25.0%.
[b]At 12% H_2O.
Source: Juliano & Villareal, 1991.

with medium to soft gel are preferred in most of South Asia (Bangladesh, India, Pakistan and Sri Lanka) for their suitability for parboiling.

Quality of rice in international markets

The quality types of rices in the international markets are basically high-quality long-grain rice, medium-quality long-grain rice, short-grain rice, parboiled rice, aromatic or fragrant rice and waxy or glutinous rice (Efferson, 1985). Each is demanded by different markets. Long-grain, higher-quality rice is sold mostly in Europe and the Near East, medium-quality long-grain rice in the deficit countries of Asia, the short-grain product in various

TABLE 23

Rice-grain apparent amylose type preferred in various rice-growing countries contributing 0.1 percent or more to total world rice production

Waxy	Low	Intermediate	High
Asia			
Laos	China (japonica)	Cambodia	Bangladesh
Thailand (north)	China-Taiwan (japonica)	China[a] (japonica)	China (indica)
	Japan	India	India
	Korea, Republic of	Indonesia	Pakistan (IR6 type)
	Nepal	Malaysia	Philippines
	Thailand (northeast)	Myanmar	Sri Lanka
		Pakistan (Basmati)	Thailand (north,
		Philippines	central, south)
		Thailand (central)	
		Viet Nam	
Outside Asia			
	Argentina	Brazil (upland)	Brazil (irrigated)
	Australia	Cuba	Colombia
	Spain	Italy	Guinea[b]
	USA (short & medium grain)	Ivory Coast	Mexico
	USSR	Liberia	Peru
		Madagascar	
		Nigeria	
		USA (long grain)	

[a]Data from China National Rice Research Institute, Hangzhou.
[b]Data from International Institute for Tropical Agriculture, Lagos, Nigeria.
Source: Juliano & Duff, 1991.

special-demand areas, high-quality parboiled rice in the Near East and Africa and the lower-quality parboiled rice in special markets in Asia and Africa. Aromatic rice is demanded mostly in the Near East. Waxy rice meets market needs in Laos, while smaller volumes go to other countries.

In the traditionally rice-consuming economies of Hong Kong and sectors of Rome, Italy, quality characteristics in major retail outlets were found to be an important consideration for retail price (Kaosa-ard and Juliano, 1989). In Hong Kong, low-amylose long-grain translucent rices are preferred, with higher head rice and softer gel consistency. In Rome, price correlated positively with chalkiness and the number of packings and negatively with gel consistency. Imported rices were more expensive than local japonica varieties, many of which were also parboiled. In Bonn, Germany, which is a traditionally non-rice-consuming market, head rice content was the only statistically important rice grain property, and level of processing, lot size and packing types were important price considerations.

Thai export rices were shown to be more variable in starch properties than United States long-grain rices, mainly intermediate-amylose, reflecting the greater heterogeneity of amylose and gelatinization temperature values among Thai varieties (Juliano, Perez and Kaosa-ard, 1990). Brokens and head rice are blended as required by the importer.

Chapter 4
Nutritional value of rice and rice diets

The gross composition of rice and its various milling fractions was given in Table 14. It shows that rice is rich in energy and is a good source of protein. Table 15 showed that rice contains a reasonable amount of thiamine, riboflavin, niacin, vitamin E and other nutrients. It does not contain any vitamin C, D or A. Because of the quantity consumed it is the principal source of energy, protein, iron, calcium, thiamine, riboflavin and niacin in Asian diets.

NUTRIENT COMPOSITION AND PROTEIN QUALITY OF RICE RELATIVE TO OTHER CEREALS

Comparison of the nutrient content of staple cereals at 14 percent moisture and higher-moisture tuber foods (Tables 24 to 27) shows a somewhat higher energy content in cereals (Table 24), but a higher ascorbic acid content in tubers (Table 25). Because tubers contain more moisture they have lower nutrient and energy density than cereals. Cassava has an extremely low protein content (Table 24) even after correction for moisture differences.

The protein level of rice is similar to those of potato and yam on a dry weight basis but is the lowest among the cereals. Rice also has the lowest dietary fibre content.

Amino acid analysis (Table 26) showed lysine to be the first limiting essential amino acid in cereal proteins, but lysine content was highest in oats and rice among cereal proteins (Eggum, 1979), (Table 26). In contrast, tuber proteins are adequate in lysine but deficient in sulphur amino acids – cysteine and methionine – particularly at high protein levels (Eppendorfer, Eggum and Bille, 1979; Food and Nutrition Research Institute, 1980).

TABLE 24

Proximate composition of cereal and tuber staple foods (per 100 g)

Food	Mois-ture (%)	Protein (g N x 6.25)	Crude fat (g)	Available carbo-hydrates (g)	Fibre (g) Dietary	Water insoluble	Lignin	Crude ash (g)	Energy (kJ)	Energy (kcal)
Brown rice	14.0	7.3	2.2	71.1	4.0	(2.7)	(0.1)	1.4	1 610	384
Wheat	14.0	10.6	1.9	61.6	10.5	(7.8)	(0.6)	1.4	1 570	375
Maize	14.0	9.8	4.9	60.9	9.0	(6.8)	(0)	1.4	1 660	396
Millet	14.0	11.5	4.7	64.6	3.7	(2.3)	(0)	1.5	1 650	395
Sorghum	14.0	8.3	3.9	57.4	13.8	(12.4)	(3.0)	2.6	1 610	384
Rye	14.0	8.7	1.5	60.9	13.1	(8.4)	(1.4)	1.8	1 570	375
Oats	14.0	9.3	5.9	63.0	5.5	(3.9)	(0)	2.3	1 640	392
Potato	77.8	2.0	0.1	15.4	2.5	(1.9)	(0)	1.0	294	70
Cassava	63.1	1.0	0.2	31.9	2.9	(2.2)	(0)	0.7	559	133
Yam	71.2	2.0	0.1	22.4	3.3	(2.6)	(0)	1.0	411	98

[a]Nitrogen-free extract by difference.
Sources: Souci, Fuchmann & Kraut, 1986; Eggum, 1969, 1977, 1979.

Whole-grain maize meal had protein quality comparable to that of wheat because of its large germ which is high in lysine-rich protein. Calculated amino acid scores based on the WHO/FAO/UNU pattern (WHO, 1985) showed tuber proteins to be superior to cereal proteins but do not take into consideration actual digestibility.

Rice has the highest protein digestibility among the staples (Table 27). Potato protein had a higher biological value than cereal proteins, consistent with its high amino acid score, but its net protein utilization (NPU) was lower than that of rice. Utilizable protein was comparable in brown rice, wheat, maize, rye, oats and potato but was lower in sorghum and higher in millet. Rice has the highest energy digestibility, probably in part because of its low dietary fibre and tannin content (Tables 24 and 26).

Cereal proteins are less digestible by children and adults than egg and milk protein, except for wheat endosperm (WHO, 1985), (Table 28). Digestibility values for cooked milled rice proteins were lower than those

TABLE 25

Vitamin and mineral content of cereal and tuber staple foods (per 100 g)

Food	Carotene (mg)	Thiamine (mg)	Riboflavin (mg)	Niacin (mg)	Ascorbic acid (mg)	Vitamin E (mg)	Iron (mg%)	Zinc[b] (mg%)
Brown rice	0	0.29	0.04	4.0	0	0.8	3	2
Wheat	0.02	0.45	0.10	3.7	0	1.4	4	3
Maize	0.37	0.32	0.10	1.9	0	1.9	3	3
Millet	0	0.63	0.33	2.0	0	0.07	7	3
Sorghum	10.0	0.33	0.13	3.4	0	0.17	9	2
Rye	0	0.66	0.25	1.3	0	1.9	9	3
Oats	0	0.60	0.14	1.3	0	0.84	4	3
Potato	0.01	0.11	0.05	1.2	17	0.06	0.8	0.3
Cassava	0.03	0.06	0.03	0.6	30	0	1.2	0.5
Yam	0.01	0.09	0.03	0.6	10	0	0.9	0.7

[a]Zinc level of cassava and yam from Bradbury & Holloway (1988).
Sources: Souci, Fuchmann & Kraut, 1986; Eggum, 1969, 1977, 1979.

for raw milled rice (almost 100 percent) when tested on growing rats but were close to the values for other cereal proteins, except for the low value for sorghum. Based on the mean true digestibility of egg, milk, cheese, meat and fish protein of 95 percent, the relative digestibility of milled rice is 93 percent (WHO, 1985). The protein of cooked rice has a lower true digestibility in humans than the protein of raw rice in growing rats (Table 28). Cooked rice protein also has a true digestibility of 89 percent in growing rats (Eggum, Resurrección and Juliano, 1977).

Nitrogen balance studies in Peruvian preschool children fed cooked cereals (Graham *et al.*, 1980; MacLean *et al.*, 1978, 1979, 1981) and potato (Lopez de Romaña *et al.*, 1980) showed the highest apparent N absorption for wheat noodles but the highest apparent N retention for peeled potato and the highest protein quality, based on apparent N retention of casein control diets, for potato and milled rice (Table 29). Utilizable protein is highest for wheat and rice. High-lysine or opaque-2 maize is inferior to milled rice in protein quality but better than normal maize. Energy digestibility, indexed

TABLE 26
Amino acid and tannin content in whole-grain cereals and tubers

Food	Lysine (g/16 g N)	Threonine (g/16 g N)	Methionine + cystine (g/16 g N)	Tryptophan (g/16 g N)	Amino acid score[a] (%)	Tannin (%)
Brown rice	3.8	3.6	3.9	1.1	66	0.4
Wheat	2.3	2.8	3.6	1.0	40	0.4
Maize	2.5	3.2	3.9	0.6	43	0.4
Millet	2.7	3.2	3.6	1.3	47	0.6
Sorghum	2.7	3.3	2.8	1.0	47	1.6
Rye	3.7	3.3	3.7	1.0	64	0.6
Oats	4.0	3.6	4.8	0.9	69	1.1
Potato	6.3	4.1	3.6	1.7	100	
Cassava	6.3	3.4	2.6	1.0	91	
Yam	6.0	3.4	2.9	1.3	100	

[a]All based on 5.8% lysine as 100%, except based on 1.1% tryptophan as 100% for cassava (WHO, 1985).
Sources: Eggum, 1969, 1977, 1979; Food and Nutrition Research Institute, 1980.

TABLE 27
Balance data of whole-grain cereals and potato in five rats

Food	True N digestibility (%)	Biological value (%)	Net protein utilization (%)	Utilizable protein (%)	Digestible energy	
					(kcal/g)	(% of total)
Brown rice	99.7	74.0	73.8	5.4	3.70	96.3
Wheat	96.0	55.0	53.0	5.6	3.24	86.4
Maize	95.0	61.0	58.0	5.7	3.21	81.0
Millet	93.0	60.0	56.0	6.4	3.44	87.2
Sorghum	84.8	59.2	50.0	4.2	3.07	79.9
Rye	77.0	77.7	59.0	5.1	3.18	85.0
Oats	84.1	70.4	59.1	5.5	2.77	70.6
Potato	82.7	80.9	66.9	5.2	–	–

Sources: Eggum, 1969, 1977, 1979.

TABLE 28

Calculated true digestibility by adults and children of various cereal proteins as compared to egg, milk and meat protein

Protein source	Mean	Digestibility relative to reference proteins
Rice, milled	88 ± 4	93
Wheat, whole	86 ± 5	90
Wheat endosperm (farina)	96 ± 4	101
Maize, whole	85 ± 6	89
Millet	79	83
Sorghum	74	78
Oatmeal	86 ± 7	90
Egg	97 ± 3	
Milk	95 ± 3	100[a]
Meat, fish	94 ± 3	

[a]Mean true digestibility of 95%.
Sources: Hopkins, 1981; WHO, 1985.

by faecal dry weight, was lowest for sorghum, probably because of its high tannin content (see Table 26).

MILLED RICE PROTEIN

The usual value assigned to the protein content of milled rice is 7 percent, based on a Kjeldahl conversion factor of 5.95. However, in nutritional studies the factor 6.25 is used to make the diets isonitrogenous with the standard proteins. The true digestibility of cooked rice protein in humans is 88 ± 4 percent (WHO, 1985), (Table 28). Its amino acid score is about 65 percent based on 5.8 percent lysine as 100 percent (WHO, 1985). The NPU of milled rice in rats is about 70 percent (Eggum and Juliano, 1973, 1975). Biological value in growing rats is about 70 percent for raw rice and about 80 percent for cooked rice (Eggum, Resurrección and Juliano, 1977).

Raw rice protein is 100 percent digestible in growing rats (Eggum and Juliano, 1973, 1975). Although cooking reduces true digestibility in

TABLE 29

Comparative protein utilization and faecal dry weight for Peruvian preschool children fed cooked cereals and potato

Cooked food	Protein (% N x 6.25)	Lysine content (g/16 g N)	Number of children	Daily N intake (mg/100 kcal)	Apparent N absorption (%)	Apparent N retention (%)	Protein quality (% of casein)	Utilizable protein (%)	Faecal dry weight (g/day)	Source
Milled rice	7.2	3.9	8	240	66.6 ± 8.6	28.6 ± 9.4	76.1	5.5	15.6 ± 2.3	MacLean et al., 1978
Wheat noodles	11.4	<2.5	9	262	81.4 ± 3.0	20.4 ± 5.8	51.0	5.8	13.3 ± 2.5	MacLean et al., 1979
Degermed maize meal (normal)	7.1	2.2	6	256	64.1 ± 11.4	15.1 ± 8.9	40.8	2.9	29.0 ± 5.0	Graham et al., 1980
Degermed maize meal (opaque-2)	6.5	3.4	6	256	69.6 ± 6.3	22.8 ± 5.5	62.0	4.0	31.0 ± 4.0	Graham et al., 1980
Whole sorghum meal	12.0	2.2	9	320	46.0 ± 21	12.0 ± 1	28.0	3.4	38.2 ± 15.3	MacLean et al., 1981
Peeled potato	5.8	~6	7	201	65.9 ± 3.7	33.9 ± 5.6	77.0	4.5	19.0 ± 4.6	Lopez de Romaña et al., 1980

growing rats to 89 percent, lysine digestibility remains close to 100 percent (Eggum, Resurrección and Juliano, 1977; Eggum, Cabrera and Juliano, 1992). Thus the NPU of cooked rice is also about 70 percent. The effects of cooking are discussed in more detail in Chapter 5.

HIGH-PROTEIN RICE

Feeding trials in growing rats and a study of growth rate data (Blackwell, Yang and Juliano, 1966), determinations of protein efficiency ratio and nitrogen growth index (Bressani, Elias and Juliano, 1971), net protein utilization studies (Eggum and Juliano, 1973, 1975; Murata, Kitagawa and Juliano, 1978) and values for relative nutritive value (Hegsted and Juliano, 1974) showed that an increase in milled rice protein from 7 to 9 percent has nutritional advantages, based on utilizable protein (protein content x protein quality), (Tables 30 and 31). The lysine content of rice protein drops only slightly with an increase in the protein content of milled rice to 10 percent and then becomes constant above 10 percent protein (Cagampang *et al.*, 1966; Juliano, Antonio and Esmama, 1973).

These rat trials were verified by isonitrogenous N balance studies in preschool children in Peru (MacLean *et al.*, 1978) and the Philippines (Roxas, Intengan and Juliano, 1979), (Table 32). Although apparent N retention was somewhat lower for the high-protein rice, the decrease was just a fraction of the increase in protein content. Short-term N balance studies also showed that with the replacement of average-protein rice (7.5 to 7.8 percent) by an equal weight of high-protein rice (11.4 to 14.5 percent) apparent N retention increased from 3.6 to 11.7 percent in adults on rice diets (Clark, Howe and Lee, 1971), from 27.7 to 29.8 percent in adults on rice/fish diets (Roxas, Intengan and Juliano, 1975) and from 21.6 to 31.6 percent in children on rice/mung bean diets (Roxas, Intengan and Juliano, 1976), (Table 33).

Long-term feeding trials in children's institutions in India and the Philippines demonstrated that replacement of average-protein (6 to 7 percent) milled rice with an equal weight of high-protein (10 percent) milled rice in children's diets improved growth, provided that other nutritional factors, such as zinc, did not become limiting (Pereira, Begum and Juliano,

TABLE 30

Relation of protein content and protein quality of milled rice based on NPU and various slope-ratio assays (weight gain) and reference proteins in growing rats

Rice protein source	Protein content (% N x 6.25)	Lysine (g/16g N)	Amino acid score[a] (%)	NPU[b] (%)	Relative nutritive value (%)			
					I[c]	II[d]	III[e]	IV[f]
Intan	6.0	4.1	70	75	78	77	82	–
Commercial	6.7	3.4	58	56	–	–	–	51
IR8	7.7	3.6	62	70	69	72	63	–
IR22	7.9	3.8	65	–	78	–	–	–
IR22	10.0	3.9	67	69	77	–	–	–
IR8	10.2	3.5	60	65	68	67	–	–
IR480-5-9	10.3	3.5	61	–	–	–	57	–	–
IR480-5-9	11.0	3.2	55	63,56	–	–	–	48
IR1103-15-8	11.6	3.6	63	71	65	–	–	–
IR58	11.8	3.5	60	68	–	–	–	–
IR480-5-9	11.8	3.3	58	64	53	–	–	–
IR480-5-9	12.3	3.3	58	–	54	–	–	–
BPI-76-1	15.2	3.2	55	66	46	60	42	–

[a]Based on 5.8% lysine as 100% (WHO, 1985).
[b]Eggum & Juliano, 1973, 1975; Murata, Kitagawa & Juliano, 1978.
[c]Based on 0, 28, 56 and 84% rice diets and lactalbumin slope as 100% (Hegsted & Juliano, 1974).
[d]Based on 0, 1, 2, 3, 4 and 5% protein diets and casein slope as 75% (Bressani, Elias & Juliano, 1971).
[e]Based on 2, 5 and 8% protein diets and casein slope as 75% (B.E. McDonald, personal communication, 1974).
[f]Based on 0, 4, 8, 12 and 15% protein diets and egg slope as 100% (Murata, Kitagawa & Juliano, 1978).

1981; Roxas, Intengan and Juliano, 1980). The absence of height or weight response by the Indian children who were without a vitamin and mineral supplement may have resulted from a deficiency in zinc and other minerals and in vitamins at the higher protein intake.

GLYCAEMIC INDEX, STARCH DIGESTIBILITY AND RESISTANT STARCH
Glycaemic index, based on the relative increase in plasma glucose within 3 hours after ingestion of carbohydrate, with white bread or glucose as 100

TABLE 31

Effect of protein content on protein quality of raw milled rice based on nitrogen balance in growing rats

Rice protein source	Protein content (% N x 6.25)	Lysine (g/16g N)	Amino acid score[a] (%)	True digestibility (%)	Biological value (%)	NPU (%)	Utilizable protein (%)
Intan	6.0	4.1	70	100.1	75.2	75.3	4.5
Commercial	6.7	3.4	58	–	–	56[b]	3.8
IR8	7.7	3.6	62	96.2	73.1	70.3	5.4
IR8	8.1	3.6	62	99.2	69.5	68.9	5.6
Perurutong	8.1	3.7	63	97.5	68.4	66.7	5.4
IR32	8.3	3.6	62	98.4	67.5	66.4	5.5
H4	9.7	3.4	58	99.2	65.7	65.2	6.3
IR8	9.9	3.4	59	98.0	69.2	67.8	6.7
IR480-5-9	9.9	3.5	60	99.8	71.0	71.0	7.0
IR22	10.0	3.9	67	98.5	69.7	68.7	6.9
IR8	10.2	3.5	60	95.4	68.4	65.2	6.7
IR2031-724-2	10.2	3.5	61	99.9	66.5	66.4	6.8
IR480-5-9	11.0	3.2	55	–	–	63,56[b]	6.9,6.2
IR480-5-9	11.2	3.4	59	100.4	66.8	67.1	7.5
IR480-5-9	11.4	3.4	58	100.6	68.4	68.8	7.8
IR1103-15-8	11.6	3.6	63	95.9	74.3	71.1	8.2
IR480-5-9	11.8	3.3	58	94.5	67.9	64.2	7.6
IR58	11.8	3.5	61	99.1	68.8	68.3	8.1
IR2153-338-3	12.2	3.6	61	98.5	69.9	68.8	8.4
IR480-5-9	13.0	3.3	57	100.1	67.7	67.8	8.8
BPI-76-1	15.2	3.2	55	94.4	70.1	66.2	10.1
IR32, destarched	18.7	4.0	70	96.8	69.0	66.8	12.5
IR480-5-9, destarched	49.4	3.3	56	94.7	65.4	61.9	30.6
IR480-5-9, gelatinized and destarched	80.2	3.6	62	92.5	73.2	67.7	54.3

[a]Based on 5.8 g lysine/16 g N as 100% (WHO, 1985).
[b]Based on carcass N analysis (Murata, Kitagawa & Juliano, 1978).
Sources: Eggum & Juliano, 1973, 1975; Eggum, Alabata & Juliano, 1981; Eggum, Juliano & Maniñgat, 1982; Eggum *et al.*, 1987; Murata, Kitagawa & Juliano, 1978; IRRI, 1976; Resurrección, Juliano & Eggum, 1978.

TABLE 32

Nitrogen balance data of high-protein and average-protein milled rice diets in male preschool children

Diet	Number of children	Protein content of rice (% N x 6.25)	Age (years)	Lysine (g/16 g N)	Daily N intake (mg/kg body wt)	Apparent N digestibility (% of intake)	Apparent N retention (% of intake)
Filipino children[a]							
High-protein rice	8	11.0	1.2-2.0	3.4	250	60.0	23.4
Low-protein rice	8	7.2	1.2-2.0	3.9	250	66.2	26.9
Peruvian children[b]							
High-protein rice	8	11.0	1.0-1.5	3.4	240	64.9	23.0
Low-protein rice	8	7.2	1.0-1.5	3.8	240	66.6	28.6

[a] First casein diet: 76.8% apparent digestibility and 30.8% apparent retention (Roxas, Intengan & Juliano, 1979).
[b] First casein diet: 86.1% apparent digestibility and 35.2% apparent retention (MacLean *et al.*, 1978).

TABLE 33

Replacement of average-protein rice by high-protein rice in various diets: effect on nitrogen balance

Subjects and diet	Number of subjects	Protein content of rice (% N x 6.25)	Daily N intake (mg/kg body wt)	Daily N retention (mg/kg body wt)	Apparent N digestibility (%)	Apparent N retention (%)	Lysine content (g/16 g N)
Adults[a]							
Low-protein rice	7	7.8	98.1	3.5	76.9	3.6	3.8
High-protein rice	6	14.5	172.7	20.2	78.0	11.7	3.1
Preschool children[b]							
Low-protein rice/fish	12	7.7	187.1	51.8	72.9	27.7	5.4
High-protein rice/fish	11	11.9	254.2	75.7	76.5	29.8	4.7
Low-protein rice/ mung bean	4	7.5	197	42	67.0	21.6	4.9
High-protein rice/ mung bean	4	11.4	256	81	75.0	31.6	4.4

[a] Clark, Howe & Lee, 1971.
[b] Milled rice/surgeon fish fillet (*Acantharus bleakeri*), (100:17 by wt), (Roxas, Intengan & Juliano, 1975); milled rice/dehulled mung bean (*Vigna radiata* [L.] Wilczek), (100:18.6 by wt), (Roxas, Intengan & Juliano, 1976).

TABLE 34

Glycaemic index of cooked milled rice and rice products of varying amylose content in normal and non-insulin-dependent diabetes mellitus (NIDDM) subjects (%)

Subjects	Waxy (0-2%)	Gruel, waxy	Low amylose (10-20%)	Intermediate amylose (20-25%)	High amylose (>25%)	Noodles, high amylose	Parboiled rice, high amylose	Reference
Normal, USA[a]	96a[e]	–	93a	81b	60c	–	–	Juliano & Goddard, 1986
Normal, Indonesia[b]	87	96	–	52	53, 70[f]	78, 82	–	Prakoso, unpublished, 1986-90
Normal & NIDDM, Canada & Philippines[b]	116c	–	–	–	61a,[g] 72ab,[g] 84-91bc[h]	58-66a[h]	66a[h]	Panlasigui, 1989
NIDDM, Thailand[b]	75a	–	71a	–	–	53-55b	–	Juliano et al., 1989a
Normal & NIDDM, Thailand[c]	(100a)	–	(87a)	–	–	–	–	Jiraratsatit et al., 1987
NIDDM, Taiwan[d]	118a	124a	111a	–	–	110a	–	Tsai et al., 1990

[a] Glycaemic index (GI) based on insulin response.
[b] GI based on glucose response, with glucose drink as 100%.
[c] The two GI values given are only relative values based on waxy rice as 100%.
[d] GI based on white bread as 100%.
[e] Letters denote Duncan's (1955) multiple range test. Values in the same column followed by the same letter are not significantly different at the 5% level.
[f] Red rice
[g] Intermediate gelatinization temperature.
[h] Low gelatinization temperature.

percent, has been used as a guide for the diets of non-insulin-dependent diabetes mellitus (NIDDM). Waxy and low-amylose rices had higher glycaemic indices than intermediate- and high-amylose rices (Goddard, Young and Marcus, 1984; Juliano and Goddard, 1986; Jiraratsatit et al., 1987; Tanchoco et al., 1990; M.I. Prakoso, 1990, personal communication), (Table 34). Processing, such as parboiling and noodle-making, tends to reduce the glycaemic index of rice, particularly that of high- and intermediate-amylose rices (Panlasigui, 1989; Wolever et al., 1986). By contrast, Tsai et al. (1990) reported that waxy rice, rice gruel, steamed rice and rice noodles had similar glycaemic indices to that of white bread in NIDDM patients. Among high-amylose rices, the low-GT, hard-gel IR42 had a higher glycaemic index than the intermediate-GT, softer-gel IR36 and IR62 (Panlasigui, 1989). By contrast, Srinivasa Rao (1970) reported that the ingestion of hard-gel IR8 resulted in a lower peak plasma glucose level than ingestion of the softer-gel Hamsa; both have high amylose and low GT.

It has been hypothesized that prolonged consumption of fibre-depleted milled rice is diabetogenic because of its low soluble fibre content (0.1 to 0.8 percent), particularly at minimum temperatures above 15°C (Trowell, 1987). Enzyme-resistant starch is reported to be affected by processing, particularly autoclaving. It acts as soluble dietary fibre in the large intestine and may have a hypocholesterolaemic effect (Englyst, Anderson and Cummings, 1983). However, reported values for enzyme-resistant starch in rice are trace to 0.3 percent (Englyst, Anderson and Cummings, 1983; Holland, Unwin and Buss, 1988). *In vitro* resistant starch values are 0 percent for raw and cooked waxy rice and less than 1 percent in raw non-waxy rice and rice noodles, but 1.5 to 1.6 percent for cooked non-waxy rice including parboiled rice. The low values may be related to the fact that rice is cooked as whole grains, which could prevent extensive starch association. A raw milled rice of amylose-extender IR36-based mutant rice had 1.8 percent *in vitro* resistant starch. Because of the importance of parboiled rice in South Asia, researchers at the National Institute of Animal Science, Foulum, Denmark are determining the enzyme-resistant starch of IR rices differing in amylose content using antibiotics to suppress hind-gut fermentation of the resistant starch (Björck *et al.*, 1987). Resistant starch was higher in cooked intermediate-GT rices than in low-GT rices and was increased by parboiling (B.O. Eggum, unpublished data). *In vitro* resistant starch obtained from cooked rices using pullulanase and ß-amylase was characterized to be essentially amylose (90 to 96 percent ß-amylolysis limits) with 55 to 65 glucose units (IRRI, 1991b), as earlier also reported for wheat and maize starch (Russell, Berry and Greenwell, 1989).

Microbial anaerobic fermentation of resistant starch in the large intestine produces lactate, short-chain fatty acids (acetate, propionate and butyrate), carbon dioxide and hydrogen. The fatty acids are absorbed from the intestinal lumen into the colonic epithelial cells and provide about 60 to 70 percent of the energy which would have been available had the carbohydrate been absorbed as glucose in the small intestine (Livesey, 1990). Thus, the complete digestion of cooked waxy and non-waxy rice starch in infants (De Vizia *et al.*, 1975; MacLean *et al.*, 1978) and of raw starch in growing rats (El-Harith, Dickerson and Walker, 1976; Eggum, Juliano and Maniñgat, 1982; Pedersen and Eggum, 1983) includes the resistant starch fermented in the large intestine or hind gut. Breath-hydrogen tests in Myanmar village children 1 to 59 months old showed a high prevalence of rice-carbohydrate malabsorption (66.5 percent), (Khin-Maung-U *et al.*, 1990a). About half of the children were in a state of current underfeeding with past malnutrition, but there was no difference between children with or without rice-carbohydrate malabsorption (Khin-Maung-U *et al.*, 1990b). Levitt *et al.* (1987) reported that rice was nearly completely absorbed by healthy adult patients and caused only a minimal increase in hydrogen excretion as compared to oats, whole wheat, maize, potatoes or baked beans.

OTHER PROPERTIES

Parboiled rice or rice powder gruel (Molla, Ahmed and Greenough, 1985), rice water (Wong, 1981; Rivera *et al.*, 1983) and extrusion-cooked rice (Tribelhorn *et al.*, 1986) have all been effectively used for the treatment of non-infectious diarrhoea since starch has a lower osmolality than glucose. Even the high concentration of 80 g rice per litre in an oral rehydration solution is drinkable by patients and is highly effective, providing four times more energy than does standard glucose oral rehydration solution (20 percent), (Molla, Ahmed and Greenough, 1985).

Consumption of cereal foods including rice has been correlated with dental caries (Bibby, 1985). Dentists agree that dental decay is the result of tooth demineralization by acids produced on the tooth surface when bacteria from carbohydrates ferment. Boiling, pressure cooking and extrusion cooking increase acid formation by starch in dental plaque. Phytate is an enamel-protective factor, together with amino acids, phosphates and lipids, etc. Refining removes caries-preventing factors from the rice foods and increases these foods' cariogenicity. The inclusion of rice bran or of a hot-water extract of rice bran in human diets has a preventive action against caries (Ventura, 1977).

There is a popular belief that some rice varieties have medicinal properties, such as the Myanmar variety Na ma tha lay. In China black rice is believed to have a body-strengthening fraction and pharmaceutical value. Thus it is known as "blood strengthening rice", "drug rice" or "(con)tributed rice" (Li and Lai, 1989). Black rice, which has a pigment level of 1 mg per 100 g rice, has 3 mg vitamin C and 0.2 mg riboflavin per 100 g and has more iron, calcium and phosphorus than non-pigmented rice. In Kerala, India, the variety Navara is believed to have medicinal properties and is used to rejuvenate the nerves in paralytic conditions: oridine, an alkaloid present in rice, has some antineurotic properties when impure (Chopra, 1933).

The anthocyanin pigments of red rice, "*tapol*", extracted with 95 percent ethanol containing 0.1 percent hydrochloric acid, are 70 percent cyanidin-3-glucoside (chrysanthemin), 12 percent peonidin-3-glucoside (oxycocci-cyanin) and two other anthocyanin pigments (Takahashi *et al.*, 1989). Pigmented brown rices were shown to have higher riboflavin but similar thiamine contents to non-pigmented IR rices (Villareal and Juliano, 1989a). The total carbohydrates and starch contents of milled red rices were reported to be lower than those of unpigmented milled rice in India (Srinivasa Rao, 1976), probably because of the higher protein content and residual phenolics with 7 percent milling in India. As brown rice, purple Perurutong had a lower NPU in growing rats (59.1 percent) than red rice (66.6 percent) and non-pigmented brown rice (66.7 to 70.6 percent) because of the extremely reduced true digestibility of its protein (72.4 percent) due to its high levels of phenolics (anthocyanin), (0.62 percent versus 0.01 to 0.25 percent), (Eggum, Alabata and Juliano, 1981). These differences are removed upon milling, which removes most of the pigments.

Varietal differences were found in cadmium (Cd) levels of brown rice grown in Tsukuba, Japan (seedlings transplanted in June 1983 and June 1985); five semi-dwarf indica rices had 24 to 74 ppb Cd, as compared to 2 to 27 ppb Cd for japonica varieties and 4 to 56 ppb Cd for non-dwarf indica varieties (Morishita *et al.*, 1987). The mean Cd content in rice from various countries ranged from 5 to 99 ppb on a wet basis, with the highest Cd content occurring in Hokuriku, Japan; daily Cd intake from rice ranged from 1 to 36 µg and was also highest in Hokuriku, but the same value (36µ) was also observed in Celibes, Indonesia, where the Cd content in rice was lower but rice intake was higher (Rivai, Koyama and Suzuki, 1990). A high cadmium content in rice was one of the major causes of an epidemic of "itai-itai" disease in Japan (Kitagishi and Yamane, 1981).

Analyses from 1979 to 1982 showed selenium (Se) deficiencies in feedstuffs in 70 percent of Chinese counties, where 80 percent of the feeds and forages analysed had less than 0.50 ppm Se (Liu, Lu and Su, 1985). The Se content of brown rice and of milled rice grown in Japan was reported to be 30 to 40 mg/g (Noda, Hirai and Dambara, 1987). Distribution of Se is 13 percent in the hull, 15 percent in bran and 72 percent in milled rice (Ferretti and Levander, 1974).

The silicon (Si) content of six milled American rices was reported to be 0.046 ± 0.030 percent (Kennedy and Schelstraete, 1975); the silicon was located mainly in the outer layer of milled rice. Energy-dispersive X-ray fluorescence spectrometry of seven IR rices indicated a mean Si content (wet basis) of 0.041 ± 0.016 percent for brown rice and 0.015 ± 0.009 percent for milled rice (Villareal, Maranville and Juliano, 1991). Colorimetric Si assay using phosphomolybdate showed that in a 7 percent protein IR32 milled rice, the Si content was 0.035 percent in the subaleurone layer (outer 9 percent), 0.014 percent in the middle endosperm (next 11 percent) and 0.009 percent in the inner endosperm (80 percent), (Juliano, 1985b), equivalent to 0.010 percent Si in the entire grain.

HYPOCHOLESTEROLAEMIC EFFECT OF RICE BRAN

In hamsters, addition to the diet of 10 percent dietary fibre from stabilized rice bran, defatted, stabilized rice bran and oat bran significantly reduced the animals' plasma cholesterol compared to the control (Kahlon *et al.*, 1990). In repeat experiments, only undefatted bran and oat bran lowered the cholesterol level (Haumann, 1989). Heat-stabilized rice bran providing 7 percent dietary fibre lowered the level of liver free cholesterol and surpassed wheat bran, when combined with 5 percent fish oil, in lowering plasma and hepatic triglycerides and hepatic lipogenesis (Topping *et al.*, 1990). Recent confirmatory human studies demonstrated the hypocholesterolaemic effect of full-fat rice bran (Gerhardt and Gallo, 1989; Nicolosi, 1990; Saunders, 1990), but limited feeding trials did not confirm the hypocholesterolaemic activity of rice bran in Japanese (brown versus milled rice), (Miyoshi *et al.*, 1987a, 1987b) or Filipino adults (Dans *et al.*, 1987).

The hypocholesterolaemic effect of oat bran is due to its high content of soluble hemicelluloses. By contrast, the hypocholesterolaemic activity of rice-bran oil in humans and rats (Raghuram, Brahmaji Rao and Rukmini, 1989) is due to the unsaponifiable matter fraction (Suzuki *et al.*, 1962; Sharma and Rukmini, 1986, 1987). Rice-bran oil lowered human blood cholesterol more effectively than did sunflower, corn and safflower oils (Suzuki *et al.*, 1962). A polysaccharide fraction in bran has also been reported to have a hypocholesterolaemic effect in rats (Vijayagopal and Kurup, 1972). The hypocholesterolaemic effect of rice-bran hemicellulose (defatted rice bran), (Ayano *et al.*, 1980) was due to the reduction of dietary cholesterol absorption from the small intestine of rats (Aoe, Ohta and Ayano, 1989).

ANTINUTRITION FACTORS

Antinutrition factors in the rice grain are concentrated in the bran fraction (embryo and aleurone layer). They include phytin (phytate), trypsin inhibitor, oryzacystatin and haemagglutinin-lectin. All except oryzacystatin have been previously reviewed (Juliano, 1985b).

All the antinutrition factors are proteins and all except phytin (phytate) are subject to heat denaturation. Phytin is located in 1- to 3-μm globoids in the aleurone and embryo protein bodies as the potassium magnesium salt. Its phosphate groups can readily complex with cations such as calcium, zinc and iron and with protein. It is heat stable and is responsible for the observed poorer mineral balance of subjects fed brown rice diets in comparison to that of subjects fed milled rice diets (Miyoshi *et al.*, 1987a, 1987b).

Trypsin inhibitor has also been isolated from rice bran and characterized (Juliano, 1985b). The partially purified inhibitor is stable at acidic and neutral pH and retained more than 50 percent of its activity after 30 minutes of incubation at 90°C at pH 2 and 7. Steaming rice bran for 6 minutes at

100°C inactivates the trypsin inhibitor, but dry heating at 100°C for up to 30 minutes is not as effective. The inhibitor distribution is 85 to 95 percent in the embryo, 5 to 10 percent in germ-free bran and none in milled rice.

Haemagglutinins (lectins) are globulins that agglutinate mammalian red blood cells and precipitate glycoconjugates or polysaccharides. The toxicity of lectins stems from their ability to bind specific carbohydrate receptor sites on the intestinal mucosal cells and to interfere with the absorption of nutrients across the intestinal wall. Rice-bran lectin binds specifically to 2-acetamido-2-deoxy-D-glucose (Poola, 1989). It is stable for 2 hours at 75°C but sharply loses activity after 30 minutes at 80°C or 2 minutes at 100°C (Ory, Bog-Hansen and Mod, 1981). Rice lectin agglutinates human A, B and O group erythrocytes. It is located in the embryo but has receptors in both rice embryo and endosperm (Miao and Tang, 1986).

Oryzacystatin is a proteinaceous (globulin) cysteine proteinase inhibitor (cystatin) from rice seed and is probably the first well-defined cystatin superfamily member of plant origin (Kondo, Abe and Arai, 1989). Incubation at pH 7 for 30 minutes at 100°C had no effect on its activity but inhibition decreased 15 percent at 110°C and 45 percent at 120°C. Oryzacystatin effectively inhibited cysteine proteinases such as papain, ficin, chymopapain and cathepsin C and had no effect on serine proteinases (trypsin, chymotrypsin and subtilisin) or carboxyl proteinase (pepsin).

An allergenic protein in rice grain, causing rice-associated atopic dermatitis in Japan, is an α-globulin and shows stable immunoreactivity (60 percent) even on heating for 60 minutes at 100°C (Matsuda *et al.*, 1988). It is present mainly in milled rice rather than in the bran. Hypoallergenic rice grains may be prepared by incubating milled rice in actinase to hydrolyse globulins in the presence of a surfactant at an alkaline pH (Watanabe *et al.*, 1990a) and washing. The color of the processed grain is improved by treatment with 0.5-N hydrochloric acid and washing with water (Watanabe *et al.*, 1990b).

PROTEIN REQUIREMENTS OF PRESCHOOL CHILDREN AND ADULTS ON RICE DIETS

The daily safe-level-of-protein requirements of preschool Filipino children consuming rice-based diets (as measured by the multilevel N balance or slope ratio method, two-thirds of nitrogen from rice) is lower for rice/milk (1.11 g/kg body wt) and rice/fish (1.18 g/kg) diets than for rice/mung bean (1.34 to 1.56 g/kg) and rice (1.44 g/kg) diets (Intengan *et al.*, 1984; Cabrera-Santiago *et al.*, 1986). True digestibilities were 70 to 78 percent. Amino acid scores of these Filipino weaning diets based on 5.8 percent lysine as 100 percent were 100 percent for rice/fish, 93 percent for rice/milk, 90 percent for rice/whole mung bean, 81 percent for rice/dehulled toasted mung bean and 60 percent for IR58 rice. The protein quality of the IR58 high-protein rice, as determined by the very short-term N balance index for three children, was 79 to 80 percent that of milk (Cabrera-Santiago *et al.*, 1986). On the basis of the safe-level-of-protein requirements for milk of 0.89 g/kg body weight (Huang, Lin and Hsu, 1980), IR58 rice had 62 percent the protein quality of milk. Toasting and dehulling of mung bean prior to boiling did not significantly improve the rice/mung bean diet because of amino acid decomposition during toasting (Eggum *et al.*, 1984). The true digestibility of rice/mung bean (2:1 by weight) diets in Thai children was 72.7 ± 6.1 percent for whole mung bean and 74.6 ± 5.9 percent for dehulled mung bean (Hussain, Tontisirin and Chaowanakarnkit, 1983).

Long-term studies in preschool children, testing protein intakes derived from short-term studies, were undertaken on two rice/fish weaning diets at 1.7 g/kg/day (Tontisirin, Ajmanwra and Valyasevi, 1984; Cabrera *et al.*, 1987). The results tend to indicate that at the protein level of 1.7 g/kg/day, the currently recommended energy intake of 100 kcal/kg/day is inadequate for growth, but further investigations using more subjects are necessary. The calculated safe level of protein intake for a 6- to 9-month-old child is 1.75 g/kg/day in developing countries, where children are exposed to infections and perhaps periodic shortages of food (WHO, 1985).

The daily safe-level-of-protein requirements for rice-based Chinese (Chen *et al.*, 1984; Huang and Lin, 1982) and Filipino (Intengan *et al.*, 1976) adult diets ranged from 1.14 to 1.18 g/kg body weight. By contrast, the safe-level-of-protein requirements for egg protein in adults were 0.89 g/kg/day (Huang and Lin, 1982) and 0.99 g/kg/day (Tontisirin, Sirichakawal and Valyasevi, 1981). The aggregated value for highly digestible, good-quality protein in healthy young men is 0.63 g/kg/day (WHO, 1985). On this basis, the rice diets provided 68 to 98 percent of the protein quality of the reference proteins. The relative NPU of rice protein in Japanese adults has been estimated by the slope ratio method as 65 percent that of egg protein (Inoue *et al.*, 1981), while NPUs of 56 percent for an egg diet and 43 percent for a Chinese rice diet have been reported (Huang and Lin, 1982).

Long-term studies (50 to 90 days) in adults, testing protein intakes derived from short-term studies, showed that protein intakes of 0.94 to 1.23 g/kg/day, at energy intakes of 37 to 63 kcal/kg/day, were adequate for Chilean, Chinese, Filipino, Korean and Thai subjects (Intengan *et àl.*, 1982; Rand, Uauy and Scrimshaw, 1984). The amino acid score for the Filipino rice diet was 100 percent (Intengan *et al.*, 1982) based on the WHO/FAO/UNU (WHO, 1985) amino acid scoring pattern for preschool children. Rice diets were calculated to be sufficient in lysine (Autret *et al.*, 1968). The calculated true digestibility of protein ranged from 80 to 87 percent for the rice diets. Based on 0.75 g of good-quality protein as the safe-level-of-protein requirement (WHO, 1985), the rice diets tested had 61 to 80 percent of the quality of the reference animal proteins. Digestibility appears to be the most important factor determining the capacity of the protein sources in a usual mixed diet to meet the protein needs of adults (WHO, 1985). Thus, because of the relatively high level of sulphur amino acids and 3.5 to 4.0 percent lysine in rice protein, milled rice complements lysine-rich, sulphur amino acid deficient legume proteins in human diets, the combination having a higher amino acid score than either rice or legume alone.

PROTEIN, ENERGY AND MINERAL UTILIZATION OF BROWN AND MILLED RICES AND RICE DIETS

FAO/WHO and the United Nations University have reviewed the research findings on energy and protein requirements using typical diets in developing countries (Torún, Young and Rand, 1981; Rand, Uauy and Scrimshaw, 1984).

Compared with milled rice, brown rice has a higher content of protein, minerals and vitamins and a higher lysine content in its protein (Resurrección, Juliano and Tanaka, 1979; Eggum, Juliano and Maniñgat, 1982), (Table 35); however, it also has a higher level of phytin, neutral detergent fibre and

TABLE 35

Composition and nutritional value of milling fractions of IR32 brown rice at 14% moisture

Rice fraction	Crude protein (%N x 6.25)	Neutral detergent fibre (%)	Crude fat (%)	Crude ash (%)	Total P (%)	Energy value (kJ/g)	Lysine (g/16 g N)	Amino acid score (%)
Brown rice	8.5	2.5	2.3	0.8	0.14	15.9	3.8	66
Undermilled rice	8.3	1.8	1.5	0.6	0.14	15.7	3.6	62
Milled rice	8.1	0.8	0.7	0.4	0.08	15.5	3.6	62
LSD	0.3	0.3	0.4	0.4	0.06	ns	0.1	

Source: Eggum, Juliano and Maniñgat, 1982.

antinutrition factors (trypsin inhibitor, oryzacystatin, haemagglutinin) in the bran fraction. Nitrogen balance studies in rats showed a slightly lower true digestibility for the protein in brown rice, but similar biological value and NPU for both brown and milled rices (Eggum, Juliano and Maniñgat, 1982), (Table 36). IR480-5-9 brown rice (10.9 percent protein) had a true digestibility of 90.8 percent, biological value of 70.8 percent and NPU of 64.2 percent (Eggum and Juliano, 1973). Digestible energy is lower in brown rice than in milled rice. Fat digestibility was 95.8 ± 0.5 percent for milled rice and 95.0 ± 0.4 percent for brown rice (Miyoshi, Okuda and Koishi, 1988). Protein digestibility was 95.3 ± 0.7 percent for milled rice and 94.1 ± 0.5 percent for brown rice.

Balance studies in rats showed digestible energy of 80.1 percent for Italian rough rice and 67.4 percent for its bran; for rough rice, N digestibility was 87.8 percent, biological value 72.6 percent and NPU 63.7 percent (Pedersen and Eggum, 1983). For IR32 rice bran (5.8 percent lysine), digestible energy was 67.4 percent, N digestibility 78.8 percent, biological value 86.6 percent and NPU 68.3 percent (Eggum, Juliano and Maniñgat, 1982). Corresponding values for rice polish (5.0 percent lysine) were 73.3 percent digestible energy, 82.5 percent apparent N digestibility, 86.3 percent biological value and 71.2 percent NPU. IR32 bran polish with 13.2 percent

TABLE 36

Balance data for milling fractions of IR32 brown rice in five growing rats[a]

Rice fraction	Digestible energy *(% of total)*	True digestibility *(% of N intake)*	Biological value *(% of digested N)*	Net protein utilization *(% of N intake)*
Brown rice	94.3b	96.9b	68.9ab	66.7a
Undermilled rice	95.5ab	97.3ab	69.7a	67.8a
Milled rice	96.6a	98.4a	67.5b	66.4a

[a] Means in the same column followed by a common letter are not significantly different at the 5% level by Duncan's (1955) multiple range test.
Source: Eggum, Juliano and Maniñgat, 1982.

protein (4.4 g lysine per 16 g N) and 15.4 percent fat, fed to growing rats, had 79.1 percent digestible energy, 85.9 percent true N digestibility, 81.1 percent biological value and 69.7 percent NPU (Eggum, *et al.*, 1984). Even with a mineral mixture in their diets, rats fed rough, brown and undermilled rices were unable to maintain their femur zinc concentration; deposition of calcium and phosphorus also appeared to be affected (Pedersen and Eggum, 1983).

Similar N balance studies for brown and milled rices were made with preschool children fed rice/casein or rice/milk (2:1 N ratio) diets (Santiago *et al.*, 1984), (Table 37). Energy absorption was better for milled rice than for brown and undermilled rice. Because of their similar N balance, the major nutritional advantage of brown rice over milled rice is its high level of B vitamins. Roxas, Loyola and Reyes (1978) reported that the true digestibility of a rice/milk diet (1:1 N source) in preschool children improved with milling: brown rice/milk, 78 ± 5 percent; undermilled rice/milk, 85 ± 5 percent; regular milled rice/milk, 87 ± 4 percent; overmilled rice/milk, 88 ± 4 percent. The brown rice diet was significantly lower in protein digestibility than the other diets.

Digestibility and balance studies in Japanese adults on brown rice and milled rice diets at low (0.5 g/kg) and standard (1.2 g/kg) protein intakes

TABLE 37

Balance data for milling fractions of IR32 brown rice in five preschool children (% of intake) [a,b]

Rice fraction	Apparent N absorbed	Apparent N retained	Apparent energy absorbed	Apparent fat absorbed
Brown rice	63a	28a	90b	93b
Undermilled rice	63a	26a	90b	96ab
Milled rice	62a	27a	93a	98a

[a] Means in the same column followed by a common letter are not significantly different at the 5% level by Duncan's (1955) multiple range test.
[b] Intake of 200 g N/kg body weight daily. First rice-casein diet (2:1 N ratio) had 77%b mean N absorbed, 33%a N absorbed, 91%ab energy absorbed and 94%b fat absorbed.
Source: Santiago *et al.*, 1984.

showed a higher energy, protein and fat digestibility for milled rice (Miyoshi *et al.*, 1986), (Table 38). Neutral detergent fibre intake was at least twice as high in the brown rice diet. These results are consistent with the data from studies on children and on rats. Studies on the same subjects showed lower apparent absorption rates for sodium, potassium and phosphorus and a lower phosphorus balance for the brown rice diet at the low protein intake (Miyoshi *et al.*, 1987b) when mineral intake was adjusted to be similar for the two diets by adding a mineral mixture. At the standard protein intake, even with higher potassium, phosphorus, calcium and magnesium levels in the brown rice diet, absorption rates of potassium and phosphorus were still significantly lower for the brown rice diet (Miyoshi *et al.*, 1987a). The contributing factor must be the high phytate level in the bran fraction (aleurone and germ) of brown rice. The results confirmed earlier balance studies comparing brown and milled rices (FAO, 1954).

TABLE 38

Digestibility and nitrogen balance data for five men on brown rice and milled rice diets at low and standard protein intake (mean ± SE)

Diet	Neutral detergent fibre intake (g/day)		Apparent energy digestibility (%)	Apparent protein digestibility (%)	True protein digestibility (%)	Apparent fat digestibility (%)	Nitrogen balance (g/day)	Transit time (hours)
	Total	From rice						
Low protein/ brown rice	13.9	13.9	89.8 ± 0.9b	48.4 ± 3.8c	63.8 ± 3.6a	76.6 ± 3.7b	-1.09 ± 0.33c	24.0 ± 1.9b
Low protein/ milled rice	5.7	5.7	96.0 ± 0.3a	68.0 ± 3.5b	83.2 ± 3.5ab	94.9 ± 0.4a	-0.71 ± 0.29bc	36.2 ± 5.2ab
Standard protein/ brown rice	31.4	23.2	89.3 ± 1.2b	72.7 ± 2.1b	80.2 ± 2.1b	74.1 ± 1.7b	-0.02 ± 0.27a	27.1 ± 0.5a
Standard protein/ milled rice	15.4	7.2	94.4 ± 0.5a	79.6 ± 1.3a	86.6 ± 1.4a	94.7 ± 0.7a	-0.38 ± 0.19ab	28.1 ± 0.6a

[a] Low protein intake, 0.5 g/kg body wt; standard protein intake, 1.2 g/kg body wt.
[b] Means in the same column followed by the same letter are not significantly different at the 5% level by Duncan's (1955) multiple range test.
Sources: Miyoshi *et al.*, 1986, 1987a, 1987b.

Chapter 5

Rice post-harvest processing, parboiling and home preparation

Considerable variation in moisture content exists among grains in the same panicle, since panicles flower and develop from top to bottom. Grain weights tend to be lower and protein content tends to be higher in the bottom branches of a panicle. Optimum moisture content for harvesting varies with the season but is usually reached about a month after flowering. Uniformity of flowering among panicles affects the percentage of immatures in the harvest crop; photosensitive rices have more synchronous flowering than non-sensitive varieties. Immature grains reduce the head rice yield and are completely chalky.

Rice is still most frequently harvested by cutting the panicle with enough stem to allow threshing by hand. The panicles are sun-dried on the bund prior to threshing by hand, treading by people or animals or processing by mechanical threshers. When threshing is delayed while the cut crop is stored in heaps, "stack burning" often results as a consequence of the anaerobic respiration of micro-organisms on the straw (70 to 80 percent moisture) and grain. Yellow or tan grains are formed when the panicle temperature reaches 60°C for a few days (Yap, Perez and Juliano, 1990). The discoloured grains have a better head rice yield and are more translucent than control grains. The mechanism seems to be non-enzymic browning (Reilly, 1990), which results in decreases in the lysine content of the protein (about 0.5 percent) and in the true digestibility to 92 percent and NPU to 61 percent (Eggum *et al.*, 1984).

Delayed harvest in rainy weather frequently leads to grain sprouting on the panicle, particularly for non-dormant japonica rices. Lodging may also cause sprouting in the panicle for non-dormant rices. The incidence of the heavy rains (cyclones) during the harvesting season in India correlates with aflatoxin contamination of the rice crop (Tulpule, Nagarajan and Bhat, 1982; Vasanthi and Bhat, 1990). Aflatoxin is also a problem in the preparation of *pinipig*, a rice product from the Philippines wherein freshly harvested waxy grains are directly steeped, without drying, prior to roasting and flaking (Food and Nutrition Research Institute, 1987).

Rough rice drying has been reviewed by Kunze and Calderwood (1985) and Mossman (1986). Solar radiation is usually used, particularly in the dry season. Drying capacity is limited in the wet season, when more rice is grown because of water availability. Flash dryers are ideal for the first drying of harvested rough rice, to decrease the moisture content to 18 to 20 percent, but no mechanical dryer has been adopted widely by Asian farmers (Habito, 1987; de Padua, 1988). Grain cracking is minimal above 18 percent moisture (Srinivas and Bhashyam, 1985; IRRI, 1991b). The initial drying will allow safe storage of the grain for up to four to five weeks before final drying. Deformation of the spherosome particles of the aleurone layer is observed during 6 to 12 months' storage in grains dried with hot air at 50°C, accompanied by a decrease in triglycerides and phospholipids (Ohta *et al.*, 1990).

Cracking occurs not during drying as sun-cracking denotes, but when the overdried grain absorbs moisture on cooling (Kunze, 1985).

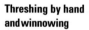

Threshing by hand and winnowing

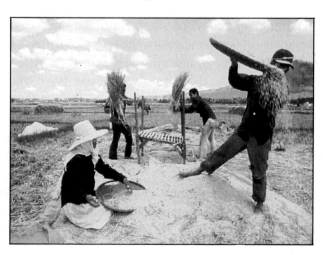

STORAGE

Storage changes, or ageing, occur particularly during the first three to four months after harvest and are also known as "after-harvest ripening" (Juliano, 1985b). The grain constituents probably equilibrate to their more stable physical form, which results in a harder, creamier-coloured grain (Yap, Perez and Juliano, 1990). After-harvest ripening is accompanied by a higher yield of total and head milled rice. Stored rice expands more in volume and yields a more flaky cooked rice with less dissolved solids in the cooking water than freshly harvested rice. In tropical Asia, aged rice is preferred and is more expensive than freshly harvested rice (Juliano, 1985b).

The exact mechanism of storage changes is not fully understood, but such changes occur in all starchy foods. In rice they occur mainly above 15°C (Juliano, 1985b). In regions where the sticky japonica rices are preferred, such as Japan and Korea, ageing in the spring and summer reduces grain quality.

The rice grain is very hygroscopic because of its starch content and equilibrates with the ambient relative humidity. The safe storage moisture content is generally considered to be 14 percent in the tropics. Storage pests (insects and micro-organisms) and rodents cause losses in both quantity and quality of the grains (Cogburn, 1985). Gross composition is not affected by storage, but vitamin content decreases progressively (Juliano, 1985b).

Rice is stored as rough rice in most of the tropics but as brown rice in Japan. Dehulling with rubber rollers minimizes bruising of the brown rice surface and improves the shelf-life of the dehulled grain. Brown rice, however, is more sensitive to environmental stress in the absence of the insulating enclosing hull and readily fissures in transit.

PARBOILING

The traditional parboiling process involves soaking rough rice overnight or longer in water at ambient temperature, followed by boiling or steaming the steeped rice at 100°C to gelatinize the starch, while the grain expands until the hull's lemma and palea start to separate (Gariboldi, 1984; Bhattacharya, 1985; Pillaiyar, 1988). The parboiled rice is then cooled and sun-dried before storage or milling.

Modern methods involve the use of a hot-water soak at 60°C (below the starch gelatinization temperature) for a few hours to reduce the incidence of aflatoxin contamination during the soaking step. Leaching of nutrients during soaking aggravates the contamination, together with the practice of recycling the soak water. Soaking sound, rough rice in water inoculated with *Aspergillus parasiticus* did not result in aflatoxin contamination of parboiled rice (Yap *et al.*, 1987), suggesting that contamination probably has to be present in the grain prior to soaking (Bandara, 1985).

Vacuum infiltration to de-aerate the grain prior to pressure soaking is applied to obtain a good-quality product, as is pressure parboiling. The parboiled product has a cream to yellow colour depending on the intensity of heat treatment. Aged rice may give a grayish parboiled rice, probably because it has a lower pH owing to the presence of free fatty acids.

Parboiling gelatinizes the starch granules and hardens the endosperm, making it translucent. Chalky grains and those with chalky back, belly or core become completely translucent on parboiling; a white core or centre indicates incomplete parboiling of the grain.

Heated-sand drying results in parboiling of the higher-moisture wet-season crop but not of the dry-season crop. Parboiling results in inward diffusion of water-soluble vitamins, in addition to partial degradation of thiamine during heat treatment, except in heated-sand drying (Padua and

Traditional batch parboiling, Bangladesh *(photo: N.H. Choudhury)*

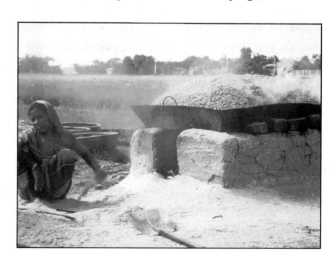

TABLE 39

Effect of parboiling method on thiamine content and protein

Treatment	Number of Samples	Degree of milling (%)		Thiamine (μg/g)				Protein (%)	
		Raw	Treated	Raw brown	Treated brown	Raw milled	Treated milled	Raw milled	Treated milled
Modified traditional (hot soak)	2	11.0	10.6	3.2	2.5	0.4	1.9	8.3	7.3
Lab. method (hot soak) 121°C 10 min	2	11.6	12.0	3.8	3.2	0.6	2.9	9.0	8.6
US commercial parboiling	3	12.2	12.6	3.9	2.8	0.5	2.1	6.6	6.2
Heated-sand drying	2	10.5	10.2	3.7	3.6	0.6	1.8	8.2	7.8
LSD (%)		0.8		0.3		0.5		0.9	

Source: Padua & Juliano, 1974.

Juliano, 1974), (Table 39). Riboflavin content is not decreased by parboiling (Grewal and Sangha, 1990). Despite the degradation of thiamine, parboiled milled rice had a higher vitamin content than raw milled rices in all parboiling procedures tested (Padua and Juliano, 1974).

Earlier results demonstrated that the water-soluble B vitamins, thiamine, riboflavin and niacin, are higher in milled parboiled rice than in milled raw rice (Kik and Williams, 1945). Oil and protein are reported to diffuse outward during parboiling, based on microscopic observations; they cannot diffuse as readily through cell walls as water-soluble vitamins, but the spherosome structure is destroyed. At similar degrees of milling, parboiled milled rice has lower protein content than raw milled rice (Table 39), but parboiled rice bran has more protein and oil than raw rice bran (Padua and Juliano, 1974). The composition of the milling fractions can be explained by a lower endosperm contamination of the bran in parboiled rice.

Parboiling results in some yellowing of the grain depending on the severity of the heat treatment. In addition, black spots diffuse to form dark brown to black regions or pecks, wherein at least 25 percent of the grain surface is coloured. Although parboiled grains are harder than raw rice, they

TABLE 40

Nutritional properties of two milled rices, raw and parboiled[a]

Rice type	Crude protein (% N x 6.25)	Lysine (g/16 g N)	Balance data in five growing rats			
			True digestibility (% of N intake)	Biological value (% of digested N)	Net protein utilization (% of N intake)	Digestible energy (% of intake)
IR480-5-9[b]						
Raw	11.2	3.4	100.4	66.8	67.1	97.0
Parboiled 10 min	10.4	3.6	94.7	70.4	66.7	–
IR8[c]						
Raw[d]	7.7	3.6	96.2	73.1	70.3	96.6
Parboiled 20 min	7.2	3.7	89.7	78.1	70.0	95.2
Parboiled 60 min	7.4	3.5	88.6	79.5	70.4	94.7
LSD (5%)[b]	0.2	0.2	0.9	1.1	1.4	0.5

[a]Parboiling done at 121°C; properties at 14% moisture content.
[b]Eggum, Resurrección & Juliano, 1977.
[c]Eggum *et al.*, 1984.
[d]Eggum & Juliano, 1973; Eggum, Alabata & Juliano, 1981.

are also susceptible to fissuring during drying, particularly below 18 percent moisture when free water becomes scarce in the grain.

Freshly parboiled rice may be milled directly with little breakage since the grains are pliable at high moisture content. Because of the damage to the spherosome structure, the bran of parboiled rice tends to agglomerate during milling and clog the sieves. In addition, greater milling pressure is required for parboiled rice because of the hardened endosperm.

Although parboiled rice is claimed to have a better shelf-life than raw rice because of the gelatinized starchy endosperm, its slightly open hull also makes it more exposed to insect attack. In addition, Asian parboiled rice is known to have aflatoxin contamination which is rarely found in raw rice (Tulpule, Nagarajan and Bhat, 1982; Vasanthi and Bhat, 1990). However, most of the aflatoxin is removed by processing.

The pressure parboiling process decreases the true digestibility of rice protein in growing rats (Eggum, Resurrección and Juliano, 1977; Eggum *et al.*, 1984), (Table 40). However, there is a compensatory increase in biological value such that net protein utilization is comparable in raw and parboiled milled rice. Prolonging the pressure parboiling from 20 to 60 minutes did not further reduce the protein digestibility of IR8 rice.

Parboiling also removes cooked rice volatiles including free fatty acids, inactivates enzymes such as lipase and lipoxygenase, kills the embryo and decomposes some antioxidants (Sowbhagya and Bhattacharya, 1976). Hence, cooked parboiled rice lacks the volatiles characteristic of freshly cooked raw rice – hydrogen sulphide, acetaldehyde and ammonia (Obata and Tanaka, 1965). The volatiles identified were mainly aldehydes and ketones (Tsugita, 1986).

Parboiled rice takes longer to cook than raw rice and may be presoaked in water to reduce the cooking time to be comparable to that of raw rice. The cooked grains are less sticky, do not clump and are resistant to disintegration; the grains are also harder. They also tend to expand more in girth rather than in length as compared to raw rice.

Most of the varieties parboiled in Bangladesh, Sri Lanka, India and Pakistan are the high-amylose rices that are common in these regions. In Thailand, both intermediate- and high-amylose rices are parboiled for export. Mainly long-grain, intermediate-amylose rice is parboiled in the United States, and intermediate- to low-amylose coarse japonica rices are parboiled in Italy.

Roasting of steeped rice grain at 250°C for 40 to 60 seconds also results in parboiling, but the product has a softer texture because the starch is immediately dried without permitting recrystallization or retrogradation of the starch gel, mainly the amylose fraction. The roasted grain is flattened or flaked with a wooden mortar and pestle, a roller flaker or an edge runner (Shankara *et al.*, 1984) and then winnowed to remove hull and germ.

PROCESSING

Dehulling of rough rice to brown rice can be carried out either manually (hand pounding) or mechanically. Mechanical hullers are of three main types: Engelberg mills, stone dehullers and rubber dehullers. Stone dehullers are still common in tropical Asia, where the surface-bruised brown rice is immediately milled with either an abrasive or friction mill. Rubber rollers are common in Japan, where brown rice is stored instead of rough rice, with a resultant space saving.

High humidity in the atmosphere during milling improves the yield of head rice. Increasing the moisture content of the grain to 14 to 16 percent by steam vapour prior to milling also improves the head rice yield and its taste (Furugori, 1985), since 14 to 16 percent is the critical moisture content range for crack susceptibility for most rice varieties (Srinivas and Bhashyam, 1985). Susceptible varieties readily crack below 16 percent moisture when exposed to higher humidity, but resistant varieties become susceptible at 14 percent moisture. Thus breakage is minimized for all varieties by tempering the grain to 16 percent moisture before milling. However, the milled rice may have to be redried to 14 percent for safe storage.

Rice mills in Asia range from a single-pass Engelberg mill to multipass systems. Manual technology involving hand pounding results in undermilled rice, which is richer in B vitamins than machine-milled rice because of incomplete removal of the bran layers. In the Engelberg or huller-type mill, dehulling and milling are performed in one step with greater grain breakage. The by-product is a coarse flour mixture of hull and bran. Using a dehuller before milling improves both the head and total milled rice yields. Slender grains require less pressure to mill than bold (i.e. thick) grains because of their thinner aleurone layer, but they are more prone to breakage during milling. In modern mills the milling operation involves several steps and bran and polish fractions are collected separately. Milling of 10 percent bran polish from brown rice by abrasive and friction mills removes all of the pericarp, seed-coat and nucellus and virtually all of the aleurone layer and embryo (Figure 2), but removes very little of the non-aleurone endosperm, except from the lateral ridges (Ellis, Villareal and Juliano, 1986).

The abrasive mill can overmill readily, as in obtaining white core rices with low protein and fat content for *sake* (Japanese rice wine) brewing.

The presence of chalky regions in the endosperm (white belly or white core) contributes to grain breakage during milling. Presumably a hetero-geneous endosperm is more susceptible to cracking since a chalky mutant

(Srinivas and Bhashyam, 1985) and waxy rice with a uniformly chalky endosperm (Khush and Juliano, 1985) give good milled head rice yield.

The term "polished rice" refers to milled rice that has gone through polishers that remove loose bran adhering to the surface of milled rice and improve its translucency. The polisher has a horizontal or vertical cylinder or cone, covered with leather strips, that gently removes loose bran as it is rotated in a working chamber made of a wire-mesh screen or a steel screen with slotted perforations.

Some rice consumers prefer a very glossy or shiny rice called coated or glazed rice. This rice is prepared by adding dry talc and a glucose solution to well-milled rice in a tumbler. The rotation of the tumbler distributes the mixture over the grain. The talc used to coat rice in Hawaii does not cause a higher incidence of stomach cancer as it is claimed to do in Japan, where talc-coating is banned (Stemmermann and Kolonel, 1978).

Innovations introduced in the Japanese rice industry include microcomputer control of milling based on the desired degree of milling or whiteness of the milled rice (Furugori, 1985; van Ruiten, 1985). Electronic colour sorting is commonly used to remove discoloured pecky grains. High-degree refining of milled rice, introduced in 1977, includes spraying a mist of moisture through the hollow shaft with the high-pressure air during milling, in combination with a uniquely designed metallic roll-type refining machine. Water is evaporated during milling and keeps the grain temperature lower than in regular milling. A germ rice milling machine introduced in 1976 that uses gentle, abrasive roll milling under very low pressure leaves the germ intact for more than 80 percent of the grains. Germ rice is well received by Japanese consumers because it is rich in thiamine, riboflavin, tocopherol, calcium and linoleic acid. Small coin-operated mills are becoming quite popular in Japan to handle the daily requirements of a family and thus minimize fat rancidity during storage.

Aflatoxin is produced mainly in the bran polish fraction of brown rice (Ilag and Juliano, 1982). Dehulling removes 50 to 70 percent of the aflatoxin of raw rice, and milling further reduces the toxin content to 20 to 35 percent (Vasanthi and Bhat, 1990). Parboiling reduces the toxin content in already infested rice by 33 to 61 percent; dehulling reduces toxins in parboiled rice further to 19 to 31 percent and milling to 7 to 28 percent. However, parboiled rice is a better substrate for aflatoxin production than raw rice, probably because parboiling makes the fat in rice more available for metabolism by *Aspergillus parasiticus* (Breckenridge and Arseculeratne, 1986).

Shelf-life is usually shortest for milled rice, followed by brown rice and then rough rice, because of fat rancidity. Fat in the surface cells of milled rice undergoes fat hydrolysis by lipase followed by lipoxygenase oxidation of the liberated free unsaturated fatty acids. With brown rice, the dehuller used is the critical factor; a rubber dehuller is preferred over a stone dehuller, to reduce surface bruises on the grain that trigger lipase action on lipids.

POST-HARVEST LOSSES

Rice losses occur at all stages of the post-harvest chain. Though quantitative losses are usually simple to assess, qualitative ones are more difficult to define and rely more on subjective judgements and cultural perceptions. Accepted figures for quantitative post-harvest losses in rice range from 10 to almost 40 percent, with the following breakdown:
- harvesting, 1 to 3 percent,
- handling, 2 to 7 percent,
- threshing, 2 to 6 percent,
- drying, 1 to 5 percent,
- storage, 2 to 6 percent,
- milling, 2 to 10 percent.

These figures, initially collected in Southeast Asia (de Padua, 1979), were later confirmed for other parts of Asia and Africa by field activities of FAO's Prevention of Food Losses (PFL) programme, among others. They have become the standard values for rice losses.

The timing of the rice harvest influences the level of losses. Depending on the variety, delay in harvesting a mature rice crop leads to lower yields because of lodging and shattering and the exposure of the ripe grain in the field to insects, birds and rodents. It also leads to post-harvest losses by lowering milling yields and recovery of head grains.

Traditional threshing techniques are a frequent cause of loss. These include beating the straws against slats through which the grain falls into tubs or buckets, trampling with feet and occasionally using a tractor or tractor-drawn roller. Quality is affected since grains might break or stones and soil become mixed with the threshed rice.

Often a considerable amount of grain is scattered around and gets eaten by poultry and household pets. However, while this quantity can be considered lost for human consumption, it becomes productive within the total household economy.

Threshed rough rice is commonly stored either in sacks or in bulk. The sacks or bags provide a means of separating varieties for specific requirements but do not provide protection against insects and rodents. Good store management, proper dunnage and adequate hygienic conditions significantly limit the losses.

On the large scale, bulk storage and controlled-atmosphere storage, if properly organized, are efficient and relatively inexpensive. However, efficient operation requires considerable capital investment and trained labour which often go beyond the single farmer's capability.

Storing rice as rough rice has advantages over storing milled rice, since the hull protects the kernel against insects and fungal attacks. This possibility depends to some extent on the local economic situation and on supply and demand for rough rice and milled rice at different times in the season.

HOME PREPARATION AND COOKING

Washing of milled rice prior to cooking is a common practice in Asia to remove bran, dust and dirt from the food, since rice is often retained in open bins and thus exposed to contamination. During washing some water-soluble nutrients are leached out and removed. Table 41 presents the washing and cooking losses of nutrients from various types of rice. It indicates that a significant amount of protein, ash, water-soluble vitamins and minerals and up to two-thirds of crude fat may be removed during washing. Marketing clean packaged rice will reduce or delete washing steps and prevent or reduce loss of nutrients during washing.

Boiling in excess water results in leaching out of water-soluble nutrients including starch and their loss when the cooking liquor is discarded. For example, 0.8 percent of the starch was removed on two washings of three

TABLE 41

Percent nutrient losses during washing and cooking in excess water

Nutrient	Washing[a]			Washing and cooking[b]	Cooking without washing[c]		
	Raw milled rice	Brown rice	Parboiled milled rice	Milled rice	Milled rice	Brown rice	Parboiled milled rice
Weight	1-3	0.3-0.4		5-9	2-6	1-2	3
Protein	2-7	0-1		2	0-7	4-6	0
Crude fat	25-65			50	36-58	2-10	27-51
Crude fiber	30						
Crude ash	49				16-25	11-19	29-38
Free sugars	60			40			
Total polysaccharides	1-2			10			
Free amino acids	15			15			
Calcium	18-26	4-5		1-25	21		
Total phosphorus	20-47	4		5			
Phytin phosphorus	44						
Iron	18-47	1-10			23		
Zinc	11			1			
Magnesium	7-70	1		1			
Potassium	20-41	5		15			
Thiamine	22-59	1-21	7-15	11	47-52		
Riboflavin	11-26	2-8	12-15	10	35-43		
Niacin	20-60	3-13	10-13	13	45-55		

[a] Kik & Williams, 1945; Cheigh *et al.*, 1977a; Tsutsumi & Shimomura, 1978; Hayakawa & Igaue, 1979; Perez *et al.*, 1987.
[b] Cheigh *et al.*, 1977a, 1977b; Perez *et al.*, 1987.
[c] El Bayâ, Nierle & Wolff, 1980.
Source: Juliano, 1985b.

milled rices, but 14.3 percent of the starch by weight was in the rice gruel after cooking for about 20 minutes in 10 weights of water (Perez *et al.*, 1987). Protein removal was 0.4 percent during washing and 0.5 percent during cooking. Boil-in-the-bag parboiled rice in perforated plastic bags makes cooking in excess water simple and convenient. In the rice cooker or optimum-water-level method, the leachate sticks to the cooked rice surface as the water gets absorbed by the rice starch. The bottom layer is more mushy than the top layer.

Increasing the proportion of brokens in milled rice from 0 to 50 percent by weight increases loss of solids on cooking of raw rice from 13 to 27 percent (Clarke, 1982). A contributing factor is the shorter cooking time of brokens: the proportionate loss from the experiment was 22 percent for large brokens and 47 percent for small brokens.

Boiling in adequate cooking water also reduces the aflatoxin content of milled rice by 50 percent (Rehana, Basappa and Sreenivasa Murthy, 1979). Pressure-cooking destroys 73 percent of the aflatoxin, and cooking with excess water destroys 82 percent.

Boiling reduces the true digestibility of milled rice protein by 10 to 15 percent but has no effect on other cereal proteins (Eggum, 1973); however, it improves the biological value of the protein such that net protein utilization in rats is not reduced notably because lysine digestibility is not reduced (Eggum, Resurrección and Juliano, 1977), (Table 42). The undigested protein, which passes out of the alimentary system as faecal protein particles, represents the lipid-rich core protein of spherical protein bodies (Tanaka *et al.*, 1978), which is poor in lysine but rich in cysteine (Tanaka *et al.*, 1978; Resurrección and Juliano, 1981), (Table 43). Mutants with reduced levels of minor sulphur-rich fractions of rice prolamin (10 and 16 kd) are being developed to improve the digestibility of the protein of cooked rice, since the minor prolamin fractions are probably in the core fraction. Parboiling further reduces protein digestibility and increases the biological value correspondingly, without any adverse effect on net protein utilization (Eggum, Resurrección and Juliano, 1977; Eggum *et al.*, 1984), (Table 40). The reported true digestibility of cooked milled rice is 88 ± 4 percent in adults and children (Hopkins, 1981), (Table 28).

Tanaka and Ogawa (1988) found greater amounts of large spherical protein bodies (PB-I) in indica rice (30 percent) than in japonica rice (20 percent), (Ogawa *et al.*, 1987) and suggested that the protein of cooked indica rice may be less digestible than that of cooked japonica rice.

TABLE 42

Mean nutritional properties of various raw and cooked, freeze-dried milled rices at 14 percent moisture

Rice type	Crude protein (% N x 6.25)	Lysine (g/16 g N)	Balance data in five growing rats						
			True digestibility (% of N intake)	Biological value (% of digested N)	Net protein utilization (% of intake)	Energy utilization[a] (% of intake)	Starch digestibility[a] (% of intake)	Lysine digestibility[a] (% of intake)	Cysteine digestibility[a] (% of intake)
IR29, IR32, IR480-5-9 [b]									
Raw	8.9	3.6	99.7	67.7	67.5	96.8	99.9	99.9	99.5
Cooked, freeze-dried	9.0	3.5	88.6	78.2	69.2	95.4	99.9	99.4	82.0
IR58 [c]									
Raw	11.8	3.5	99.1	68.8	68.3	97.0	–	–	–
Cooked, freeze-dried [d]	12.7	3.5	85.8	73.7	63.2	92.5	–	–	–

[a] IR29 and IR480-5-9 only
[b] Eggum, Resurrección & Juliano, 1977.
[c] IRRI, 1984a.
[d] Eggum et al., 1987.

TABLE 43

Properties of whole and pepsin-treated cooked IR480-5-9 and IR58 milled-rice protein bodies[a]

Protein bodies	Weight recovery (% of milled rice)	Crude protein (% N x 5.95)	Lysine (g/16.8 g N)	Cysteine (g/16.8 g N)	Methionine (g/16.8 g N)	Crude lipids (%)	Neutral lipid: glycolipid: phospholipid ratio	Carbohydrate (% anhydro-glucose)	Polypeptide molecular mass (kd)
Whole protein bodies									
IR480-5-9	13.0	79.1	4.0	2.6	3.1	9.5	92:5:3	–	38,25,16
IR58	12.0	81.3	4.0	3.0	2.2	7.4	–	5.3	38,25,16
Pepsin-treated protein bodies									
IR480-5-9 (1X)[b]	4.6	62.4	1.3	4.6	4.8	22.0	92:5:3	–	16
IR58 (1X)	4.3	60.3	1.7	4.1	2.6	–	–	–	16
IR58 (2X)	3.0	51.6	0.8	3.1	3.3	21.4	–	21.3	16

[a]Protein content of 10.5% for IR480-5-9 and 11.8% for IR58 milled rice.
[b]Number of pepsin treatments.
Sources: Resurrección & Juliano, 1981; Resurrección *et al.*, 1992.

However, Tanaka, Hayashida and Hongo (1975) and Tanaka *et al.* (1978) reported similar *in vitro* digestibilities for protein bodies from japonica and indica rices.

The low lysine content in the protein of pepsin-treated protein bodies and faecal protein particles (Tanaka *et al.*, 1978) explains the retention of the high lysine digestibility of rice protein on cooking. Its high cysteine content also explains why cysteine has the lowest digestibility among the amino acids of rice proteins (Tanaka *et al.*, 1978).

The FAO/WHO method of protein quality evaluation is based on the amino acid score times true digestibility (TD) in rats (FAO, 1990c). Application of this method to the cooked composite rice diets of preschool and adult Filipinos and to their cooked rice component (Eggum, Cabrera and Juliano, 1992) gave protein quality values 6 to 8 percent lower (56 percent for rice and 89 and 80 percent for the two rice diets) than those based on lysine digestibility (62 percent and 95 and 88 percent, respectively). TD was 88 to 90 percent for the three samples, and lysine digestibility was 95 to 96 percent for the rice diets and 100 percent for cooked rice. Milled rice had higher digestible energy and protein but lower biological value and net protein utilization (NPU) than the rice diets. Amino acid scores and protein quality of the rice diets were as high or higher than their NPU, but the NPU of milled rice was higher than its amino acid score and protein quality. Thus, the new method will underestimate the protein quality of cooked rice, but not that of raw rice with 100 percent protein and lysine digestibilities in growing rats (Eggum, Resurrección and Juliano, 1977).

Chapter 6
Major processed rice products

Consumption of processed rice products is probably highest in Japan, where it accounted for about 9.5 percent of total rice consumption in 1987 (4.8 percent *sake*, 1.0 percent *miso*, 2.0 percent crackers, 1.0 percent flour and 0.4 percent each packaged rice cake and boiled rice products), (Hirao, 1990). In comparison, processed rice products have accounted for about 2 percent of rice consumption in the Philippines (Food and Nutrition Research Institute, 1984), about 1 percent (as noodles) in Malaysia (FAO, 1985) and over 1 percent in Thailand (Maneepun, 1987).

In countries such as Japan and the Republic of Korea where per caput consumption of boiled rice is decreasing, maintenance of rice consumption is being pursued through the development of new products and the improvement of traditional products in order to maintain total rice production. Japan has the widest range of convenience rice products, including automated cooking equipment for catering (Juliano and Sakurai, 1985). Many national programmes are also looking into the improvement of the quality and shelf-life of traditional rice products (FAO, 1985). Japan's super-rice programme will incorporate selected preferred characteristics of foreign rice into the new Japanese rices (Yokoo, 1990).

Processed rice products may be derived from rough rice, brown rice, milled rice, cooked rice, brokens, dry-milled flour, wet-milled flour or rice starch (Juliano and Hicks, 1993), (Figure 5). The nutrient composition of some rice products is summarized in Table 44.

PRECOOKED AND QUICK-COOKING RICES
Precooked rice is used for rice-based convenience food products in which non-rice ingredients are packed separately and mixed only during heating. Retort rice in Japan is made by hermetically sealing cooked non-waxy and

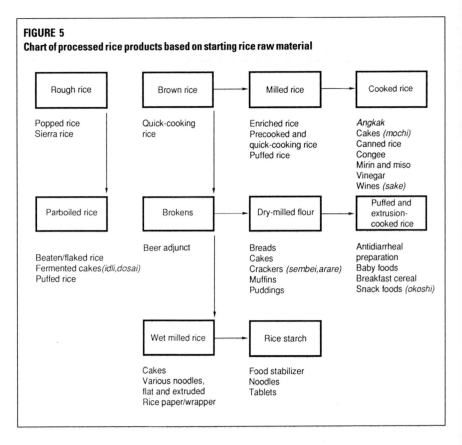

FIGURE 5
Chart of processed rice products based on starting rice raw material

waxy rice in laminated plastic or aluminium-laminated plastic pouches and pasteurizing at 120°C under pressure (Juliano and Sakurai, 1985; Tani, 1985). Steamed waxy rice with red beans accounts for 80 percent of retort rice in Japan, with an annual production of 8 030 t in 1983 (Tani, 1985) and 4 264 t in 1986 (Iwasaki, 1987). An aluminium-laminated plastic pouch is warmed directly in hot water for 10 to 15 minutes, while plastic pouches may be punctured and heated in a microwave oven for 1 to 2 minutes.

Frozen cooked rice packed in airtight plastic pouches had a production figure of 10 841 t in 1983 in Japan (Tani, 1985); 22 575 t were produced in 1986 (Iwasaki, 1987). Deep freezing without dehydration is the best condition for keeping cooked rice from retrograding (hardening). Frozen

TABLE 44

Nutrient composition per 100 g of selected rice products

Product	Moisture (g)	Food energy (kcal)	Protein (g)	Thiamine (mg)	Ribo-flavin (mg)	Niacin (mg)
Instant rice, US	9.6	362	7.5	0.44	–	3.5
Rice, granulated, US[a]	7.4	383	6.0	0.42	0.11	5.8
Kaset rice-soybean infant food, Thailand[a]	5.2	401	11.0	0.2	0.4	1.0
Baby cereals, rice-based, UK[a]	4.9	386	10.9	1.60	1.20	23.0
Am, thin rice gruel, Philippines	95.9	17	0.1	0.02	0.02	0.4
Rice gruel, Philippines	91.5	30	0.6	0.01	0.01	0.1
Arroz caldo, rice gruel, Philippines	83.8	63	2.0	0.02	0.03	0.4
Bihon, rice noodles, Philippines	12.4	364	5.0	trace	0.01	0.2
Fermented rice/black gram *idli*, India	45.0	220	7.6	0.32	0.30	0.9
Puto, fermented rice cake, Philippines	46.6	214	2.8	0.01	0.01	0.4
Chinese waxy rice cake, UK	29.8	290	3.5	trace	0.02	0.9
Bibingka, rice cake, Philippines	41.5	234	3.6	0.12	0.05	0.6
Waxy rice *bibingka*, Philippines	36.8	256	2.8	0.03	0.01	1.1
Kutsinta, rice cake with lye, Philippines	58.9	167	1.4	trace	0.01	0.2
Suman, waxy rice cake with lye, Philippines	52.3	191	3.2	trace	0.02	0.5
Suman sa ibos, waxy rice cake with coconut milk, Philippines	57.5	171	3.1	0.01	0.01	0.3
Tikoy, waxy rice cake, Philippines	37.7	250	2.5	0.02	0.02	0.4
Puto bumbong, purple waxy rice cake, Philippines	38.5	251	3.5	0.03	0.01	0.4
Palitaw, waxy rice preparation, Philippines	51.8	206	2.6	0.04	0.02	0.7
Kalamay, waxy rice preparation with coconut syrup, Philippines	48.2	208	2.7	0.01	0.01	0.3
Espasol, waxy rice product, Philippines	25.8	312	4.0	0.06	0.04	1.1
Tamales, rice flour preparation, Philippines	75.2	100	1.3	0.01	0.02	0.4
Puffed rice, US[a]	3.7	399	6.0	0.44	0.04	4.4
Puffed rice, non-waxy, sweetened	5.6	385	4.5	0.01	0.14	1.6

(continued)

TABLE 44 (continued)

Product	Moisture (g)	Food energy (kcal)	Protein (g)	Thiamine (mg)	Ribo-flavin (mg)	Niacin (mg)
Puffed rice, presweetened, with cocoa, US[a]	3.4	401	4.5	0.42	0.06	6.3
Pinipig, flattened parboiled waxy rice, puffed, Philippines	3.3	392	3.1	trace	0.04	2.0
Puto seko, toasted rice bread, Philippines	4.8	388	6.0	0.06	0.02	0.5
Rice pudding, canned, UK	77.6	89	3.4	0.03	0.14	0.2
Chicken with rice soup, condensed, US	89.6	39	2.6	trace	0.02	0.6
Japanese *sake* rice wine, 32 proof	78.4	134	0.5	0	0	0
Chinese rice wine, 34 proof	79.1	132	0	trace	0.01	0.12
Rice flour, UK	11.8	366	6.4	0.10	0.05	2.1
Rice starch	13.8	343	0.8	–	–	–

[a] With added vitamins and minerals.
Sources: Food and Nutrition Research Institute, 1980; Watt and Merrill, 1963; Luh and Bhumiratana, 1980; Holland, Unwin and Buss, 1988.

rice produced in cooking centres is delivered to chain restaurants where it is heated in microwave ovens and served to customers.

Quick-cooking rices are those that require significantly less cooking time than raw milled rices (15 to 25 minutes). Various methods are employed to fissure raw rice or to dry cooked rice to produce a porous structure. Dry-heat methods include heating milled and brown rice with 57 to 82°C air for 10 to 30 minutes or with 272°C air for 17.5 seconds to fissure the grain. Japanese companies heat brown rice in a countercurrent hot air stream at 105 to 130°C for 30 minutes and quickly cool it to below 30°C (Juliano and Sakurai, 1985). Parboiled brown rice may be made quick-cooking by scouring about 1 percent by weight of the pericarp to remove the outer water-impervious layer (Desikachar, Raghavandra Rao and Ananthachar, 1965). Precooked quick-cooking rice processes include soak-boil-steam-dry, gelatinize-dry-puff, gelatinize-roll or bump-dry, freeze-thaw, gun puff, freeze-dry and chemical treatments (Roberts, 1972).

Pregelatinized or "alpha" rice production in Japan was 13 900 t in 1983 (Tani, 1985) and 14 500 t in 1986 (Iwasaki, 1987). Cooked rice is quickly dried by heated air to fix the starch in an amorphous state at about 8 percent moisture. Gelatinized rice is used as an emergency food and as rations in ships and mountain climbing because of its long shelf-life (three years), (Imai, 1990) and light weight (Juliano and Sakurai, 1985). It is consumed after hydration, cooking or warming for about 10 minutes and standing for about 15 minutes. Freeze-dried rice reconstituted by adding hot water to it best approximates cooked rice. Japanese instant rice gruel is prepared from pregelatinized brown-rice flour or flattened grains by adding hot water or cooking over low heat for several minutes and may be used as a weaning food.

In Taiwan Province (China), two kinds of dried cooked rice are produced commercially. One is a Cantonese-style rice congee made from non-waxy (low-amylose) milled-rice brokens, washed, ground in a hammer mill with a 5-mm screen, precooked with six times the volume of water, drum-dried for 3 minutes with a steam pressure of 5 kg/cm^2 and a clearance of 1.5 mm, flaked, mixed with dried cooked meat, vegetables, salt, monosodium glutamate and other flavourings and packed in pouches. The other product is *guo-ba*, a thin block of dried cooked waxy rice. Waxy rice is washed, soaked, cooked in a rice cooker, hand-spread in a thin uniform 0.6 cm layer on teflon-coated perforated trays, baked over a flame at 135°C for 40 minutes or at 165°C for 15 minutes, cut into 6 x 6 cm blocks and sun-dried to about 12 percent moisture. The *guo-ba* may be packaged for future use, may be further flavoured and fried, may be used as a ready-to-eat snack or breakfast food or may be added as an ingredient in cooked dishes. Both products involve spreading the cooked rice into layers by hand, which is both time consuming and a potential source of contamination.

Dry precooked rice cereal is produced by preparing and cooking a cereal slurry, which is then dried in a double-drum atmospheric dryer, flaked and packed (Brockington and Kelly, 1972). The slurry solids, drum speed and temperature and spacing between drums are carefully controlled. Hydrated precooked and ready-to-eat infant foods must have the right consistency, soft enough to be swallowed easily but thick enough to feed without spilling. Malt and fungal α-amylase may be added to control the quantity of liquid required to reconstitute the dried cereal and to sweeten it by partial hydrolysis of the starch. Rice-based weaning foods are popular in Southeast Asia, such as the Kaset extrusion-cooked rice and full-fat soybean formulation (Luh and Bhumiratana, 1980). Heat-sensitive ingredients such as milk are preferably added after extrusion, to avoid lysine and cysteine degradation of the protein.

NOODLES

Flat and extruded round noodles and rice paper are traditionally prepared from wet-milled flour that has been ground using either a stone or a metal mill. The starting material is brokens with a low fat content, preferably freshly milled from aged rice with a high apparent amylose content and a hard gel consistency.

To make flat rice noodles, a wet-milled rice batter with a consistency of 42 percent rice by weight is placed on a noodle-making machine until the drum is half immersed. The smooth drum is then slowly rotated. The adhering batter is scraped off by a stainless steel sheet set at about a 45° angle and flows onto a moving taut cotton or stainless-steel conveyor belt that carries it into a steam tunnel for 3 minutes for gelatinization (to 62 percent moisture), (Juliano and Sakurai, 1985; Maneepun, 1987). The sheet dips

Extruded rice noodle
factory based on
continuous process,
Thailand
(photo: M.H. Cosgriff)

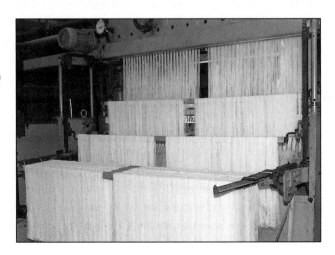

momentarily into peanut oil before it is folded and cut into appropriate sheets (50 x 50 cm) for direct sale as fresh noodle. Very little starch degradation occurs in the process.

Rice paper and egg roll wrapper are also prepared from wet-milled high-amylose rice batter in Viet Nam, Thailand and Taiwan. A measured volume of rice batter, with the proper consistency, is poured with a flat shallow ladle over taut cheesecloth on top of a steamer. The batter is spread over the whole surface by a circular motion of the ladle and steamed until gelatinized. The sheet is then removed with a rolling motion onto a rolling pin and unrolled onto a slotted-bamboo drying tray. Rice paper is thinner than egg roll wrapper and is used as translucent edible candy wrapper. The egg roll wrapper may have some added salt.

A cooked rice slurry with added food colours is poured onto various leaf surfaces, dried and peeled off and used as colourful decorations for homes during the annual May 15 festival at Lucban, Quezon in the Philippines. These edible decorations, *kiping*, retain the vein patterns of the various leaves on to which they are poured.

Traditionally, extruded noodles (*bihon, bijon, bifun, mehon* or *vermicelli*) are prepared from aged high-amylose brokens by wet-milling the steeped rice, kneading it into fist-sized balls, surface-gelatinizing the flour balls (about 500 g) in a boiling water bath until they float, remixing, extruding through a hydraulic press with a die, subjecting the extruded noodles to heat treatment for surface gelatinization, soaking in cold water and sun-drying in racks (Juliano and Sakurai, 1985). Machines in Thailand knead the flour into cylinders that are steamed in portable racks and mixed mechanically into the extruder. Extruders may also be used to cook and knead premoistened dry-milled flour and then extrude it as noodle at the end of the barrel. Considerable starch degradation occurs during extrusion, such that the gel consistency changes from hard to soft. Protein quality deteriorates very little.

Fermented extruded fresh rice noodle is quite popular in Thailand. Brokens are soaked for three days for fermentation, which reduces the pH from 7 to 3.5, with *Lactobacillus* spp. and *Streptococcus* spp. (Maneepun, 1987) and are then processed in the same manner as the unfermented noodle.

Protein decreases from 1.54 percent after one day of fermentation to 1.14 percent after three days at 70 percent moisture.

During wet milling, water-soluble nutrients and damaged starch are lost in the filtration step. Nutrient losses include vitamins, minerals, free sugars and amino acids, water-soluble polysaccharides and protein (albumin) and fat. The wastewater poses a pollution problem. Many Philippine extruded noodle plants use maize starch to minimize the pollution, but maize starch noodle has lower nutritional value (<1 percent protein) than rice noodle.

RICE CAKES, FERMENTED RICE CAKES AND PUDDINGS

Wet-milled non-waxy or waxy rice flour may be kneaded with water and converted to sweetened rice cake by adding sugar and other ingredients before steaming. A yeast-fermented steamed rice cake (*puto*) is produced in the Philippines, for which aged, intermediate-amylose rice yields the greatest volume expansion and optimum softness (Perez and Juliano, 1988). *Nenkau* is a traditional Chinese rice cake and is basically of three types: a sweetened cake made of waxy rice and sugar; a savoury cake with radish, made from high-amylose rice mixed with crushed radish; and a fermented rice cake, made of fermented rice dough of high-amylose rice and sugar.

Idli (rice dumpling) and *dosai* (rice pancake) are prepared in India from a mixture of parboiled milled rice and black gram (*Phaseolus mungo*), about 3:1 by weight, typically as breakfast foods (Hesseltine, 1979; Steinkraus, 1983). Rice and decorticated black gram are separately washed, soaked 5 to 10 hours in 1.5 to 2.2 times by weight of water and wet-milled separately to give a coarse (0.6 mm) rice flour and a smooth, gelatinous gram paste. The flour and paste are mixed together with 0.8 percent salt and the thick batter is fermented overnight, steamed (*idli*) or fried (*dosai*) and served hot. Ingredients added to *idli* for flavour include cashew nut, ghee, pepper, ginger, sour buttermilk and yeast. *Dosai* usually contains less black gram. The batter quality of *idli* is attributed to the globulin protein and the arabinogalactan of the black gram (Susheelamma and Rao, 1979). Parboiled high-amylose rices are suitable for *idli*. During fermentation, B vitamins and vitamin C increase (Soni and Sandhu, 1989) and phytate is about 50 percent hydrolysed.

A Philippine rice cake, *bibingka*, is made from non-waxy and waxy rice flour (wet-milled) with sugar and coconut milk, baked in a banana-leaf lined pan in a charcoal stove with live charcoal on top until brown. Another rice cake, *puto kutsinta*, is an unleavened cake textured like a stiff pudding and is prepared from wet-milled rice flour with sugar and lye.

Japanese rice cake or paste (*mochi*) is traditionally prepared from waxy milled rice by washing the milled rice, steaming at 100°C for about 15 minutes to a 40 percent moisture content, grinding (kneading or using a mortar and pestle), packing in plastic film, pasteurizing for 20 minutes at 80°C and cooling (Juliano and Sakurai, 1985). Recently, gelatinized waxy-rice flour has been directly manufactured by extrusion cooking; it has diverse applications, including *mochi*. *Mochi* is usually sliced into pieces (such as cubes), toasted and seasoned with soy sauce or wrapped and eaten as a snack. Preferred waxy rices have a final starch GT of 66 to 69°C (Palmiano and Juliano, 1972). Ready-to-eat *mochi* is pasteurized under 95°C in packaged containers (Tani, 1985). Annual consumption in Japan was 42 000 t in 1983 and 52 305 t in 1986 (Iwasaki, 1987).

Traditional Philippine waxy-rice snack foods or desserts include rice cakes (*suman*) made from milled rice. *Suman sa antala* and *suman sa ibos* are cooked with coconut milk and salt. *Suman sa antala* is wrapped in heat-wilted banana leaves and steamed for 30 to 35 minutes, but for *suman sa ibos* the waxy rice/coconut milk mixture is packed loosely into nipa or palm leaves (*ibos*) and boiled for 2 hours or until done. In *suman sa lihiya*, the steeped waxy rice is treated with lye, wrapped in banana leaves and boiled for 2 hours or until done. *Suman sa ibos* is usually served with sugar, while *suman sa lihiya* is served with grated coconut and sugar. Low-GT waxy rices are preferred for these cakes. Wet-milled purple waxy rice is added to waxy rice in preparing *puto bumbong*, wherein the rice flour is cooked by steaming in bamboo cylinders. Food colouring is now used to obtain the purple colour of the product, which is also eaten with grated coconut and sugar. *Palitaw* is made from a flattened wet-milled batter of waxy rice dropped into boiling water; after the cakes float they are dropped into cold water to prevent them from sticking to each other. They are drained and served with grated coconut and pounded sesame seeds. *Espasol* is made from coconut milk and sugar syrup to which cooked waxy rice is added, followed by toasted and powdered waxy rice. The paste is rolled with a rolling pin and cut into various shapes. Rice powder is sprinkled over the paste to prevent sticking. *Tamales* contains toasted, ground rice and a mixture of peanuts, sugar, spices and meat which is cooked until thick enough to hold its shape. It is then wrapped in banana leaves and steamed for 2 hours.

The Japanese rice pudding *uiro* consists of waxy rice flour, cornstarch, sugar, water and flavourings that are mixed and steamed for 60 minutes at 100°C and served with sweet bean curd, green tea, coffee, cherries and other fruits (Juliano and Sakurai, 1985). Low-amylose, short- to medium-grain rices are used in preparing Chinese rice pudding (Li and Luh, 1980). The rice is cooked in boiling water, strained and mixed with milk before the completion of cooking. Egg yolk, sugar, vanilla and light cream are added together with a variety of fruit combinations. Canned rice pudding in a milk base with added fruit has been available in Australia and the United Kingdom for more than two decades.

EXPANDED (PUFFED, POPPED) RICE PRODUCTS

Puffed and popped rices are traditional breakfast cereals and snack foods (Juliano and Sakurai, 1985). Raw rice is traditionally popped by heating rough rice (13 to 17 percent moisture) at about 240°C for 30 to 35 seconds or at 275°C for 40 to 45 seconds or in an oil bath at 215 to 230°C. The hull contributes to pressure retention before popping as evidenced by the lower popping percentage of brown rice. Good popping varieties have a tight hull and a significant clearance between hull and brown rice and when freshly harvested are free of grain fissures (Srinivas and Desikachar, 1973). Tightness of hull, grain hardness and degree of translucency could explain 80 percent of the variation in popping expansion among 25 rice varieties (Murugesan and Bhattacharya, 1991).

Flaked or beaten brown rice and parboiled milled rice may be converted to puffed rice by heating in hot air or roasting in hot sand (Juliano and Sakurai, 1985; Villareal and Juliano, 1987). With normal parboiled milled rice, puffed volume is directly proportional to the severity of parboiling (equilibrium water content of steeped grain prior to parboiling) and is highest for waxy rice (Antonio and Juliano, 1973). Puffed waxy and low-amylose rices tend to have a higher puffed volume than intermediate- to high-amylose rices only when grains are incompletely parboiled or cooked before oil puffing (Villareal and Juliano, 1987). However, with increasing temperature and period of roasting of rough rice, high-amylose rice (specifically 27 percent) gives the maximum puffed volume for roasted beaten rice (Chinnaswamy and Bhattacharya, 1984). Puffed non-waxy rice and flattened waxy rice are caramelized and moulded and are common snack foods in the Philippines. A typical Japanese rice cake, *okoshi*, is made of puffed broken rice mixed and moulded with millet jelly, sugar and flavouring.

Gun-puffing of moist milled rice may be considered as puffing rather than popping since the grains are gelatinized prior to expansion. The expansion ratio was higher for waxy milled rice than for non-waxy rice (Villareal and Juliano, 1987). The expansion ratio for gun-puffed milled rice or oil-puffed parboiled or boiled milled rice correlated negatively with protein content, except for those rices parboiled at zero steam pressure before oil-puffing.

Continuous explosion-puffing of brown rice, developed in Japan in 1971, uses a long heating pipe wherein grains are dispersed and conveyed by a high-velocity stream of superheated steam (Sagara, 1988). After the rice has been heated and dried within 3 to 10 seconds, it is discharged into the atmosphere through a rotary valve to explosion-puff. A brown rice expansion ratio of 5.4 is obtained at 6 kg/cm^2 pressure and an outlet steam temperature of 200ºC. The puffed product has a starch digestibility of 94 percent after 15 minutes of boiling. Thiamine is not destroyed at 200ºC or lower but is completely destroyed at an outlet steam temperature of 240ºC (Sagara, 1988).

In developed countries, dry rice breakfast cereals include rice flakes, oven-puffed, gun-puffed or extruder-puffed rice, shredded rice cereal and multigrain cereals (Brockington and Kelly, 1972; Luh and Bhumiratana, 1980). These are of the ready-to-eat type in which the rice starch provides texture-modifying properties and rice also imparts its own special flavour. Among the important properties of a ready-to-eat cereal is "bowl life", or the ability to retain its texture and crispness in milk while being eaten.

Moisture-proof packaging is critical for optimum shelf-life. While low-amylose, low-GT rices are used for breakfast cereals in the United States, intermediate- and high-amylose rices are used in the Philippines, but the degree of cooking must be controlled to obtain an acceptable puffed volume from the grain. Most cereals are enriched with B vitamins and with minerals, particularly iron.

BAKED RICE PRODUCTS

For those suffering from coeliac disease, a yeast-leavened bread of 100 percent rice flour has been successfully developed, consisting of 100 parts rice flour, 75 parts water, 7.5 parts sugar, 6 parts oil, 3 parts fresh compressed yeast, 3 parts hydroxypropyl methylcellulose and 2 parts salt (Bean and Nishita, 1985). Although all non-waxy rices produce breads of equivalent appearance, only low-amylose, low-GT rices give a soft-textured crumb. Intermediate-amylose, intermediate-GT rices give sandy, dry crumb characteristics. However, among low-GT rices low-amylose rice gave a lower loaf volume than did intermediate- and high-amylose rices (IRRI, 1976). Wet-milled flour gave a better texture than dry-milled flour. An extended shelf-life should improve the popularity of this product.

A medium-grain low-amylose rice flour:waxy rice flour ratio of 3:1 in place of wheat flour produced satisfactory muffins for gluten-sensitive individuals (Stucy Johnson, 1988).

For bread baking in Japan, 10 to 20 percent rice flour is generally mixed with wheat flour as a diluent, depending on the gluten strength of the wheat flour (Tani, 1985). A recent Japanese formulation consisted of 60 percent rice flour, 30 percent wheat flour and 10 percent vital gluten. Similar dilutions of wheat flour with rice flour and other starchy flours have been developed for bread-making in several countries, but the GT of the starch should preferably be low (<70°C), (Bean and Nishita, 1985).

Rice flour has also been used in making a Pakistani bread similar to *roti,* the flat unleavened bread commonly made from wheat flour (Juliano and Sakurai, 1985). The preferred bread, similar to a wheat *chapatti,* is puffed, semi-light, flexible, uniformly round and firm, but not rough. Red rices, such as Dwarf Red Gunja, are preferred in some Sind villages for Pakistani rice bread. Rice flour may also be added to wheat flour in a proportion of up to 15 percent; 21 percent rice flour in *chapatti* results in a still acceptable but difficult-to-fold texture.

Fresh pregelatinized starch is used for the preparation of wheatless bread; the starch (16 percent by weight) acts as a binder in place of gluten, as in extruded rice noodles (Satin, 1988). The method is applicable to rice flour, but the crust properties are not as good as those of wheat bread and have to be improved. Dry, pregelatinized rice flour may possibly be used to produce this bread faster without any problem of incomplete starch gelatinization during baking in the presence of sucrose.

A layer-cake formula containing 100 percent rice flour was also developed for wheat-free diets (Bean and Nishita, 1985). It consists of 100 parts rice flour, 80 parts sugar, 15 parts oil and 5 to 7 parts double-acting baking powder. Low-amylose, low-GT rices are preferred for this formula; intermediate-amylose, intermediate-GT rices give a sandy, dry texture. A high sucrose level increases starch GT; thus in 50 percent sucrose low-GT rices have a GT of 80°C while intermediate-GT rices have a GT of 92°C. When the sucrose level is reduced to give a GT of 80°C for the intermediate-GT rice, the volume and contour of the cakes improve, but the sandy texture remains. Hydrating the rice flour by intense mixing of the flour and water and folding of the hydrated mixture improve the texture and volume of the cake (Perez and Juliano, 1988).

Baked Japanese rice cakes or rice crackers include *senbei* and *arare*. *Arare* is a cracker made from boiled waxy rice pounded into rice cake, stored at 2 to 5°C for two to three days to harden, cut, dried to 20 percent moisture at 45 to 75°C and baked. *Senbei* is a cracker-like snack made of cooked non-waxy rice flour kneaded and rolled into sheets, cut, dried at 70 to 75°C to 20 percent moisture, tempered for 10 to 20 hours at room temperature, redried at 70 to 75°C to 10 to 12 percent moisture and baked at 200 to 260°C, without the cooling treatment. *Arare* expands more during baking, has a soft texture and dissolves easily in the mouth. *Senbei* is harder and rougher. Sesame seeds, pieces of dried seaweed, peanuts, pulverized shrimp, cheese or spices may be mixed with the rice dough as desired. Extruder-type kneaders are used for mixing the gelatinized rice. Rice cracker production in Japan in 1983 was 103 000 t of *arare* and 118 000 t of *senbei* (Tani, 1985) and in 1987 was equivalent to 215 000 t of brown rice (Hirao, 1990).

Non-waxy rice cakes or crackers (*xianggao*) are prepared from both low- and high-amylose rices in China. The high-amylose cake is harder, whiter and more crispy than the low-amylose cake. A similar rice product made in the Philippines from intermediate- to high-amylose rice is called *puto seko*. These crackers break readily on handling.

CANNED RICE

In the United States, the preferred canned rice product is white, with separate non-cohesive grains, minimal longitudinal splitting and fraying of edges and ends and a clear canning liquor (Burns and Gerdes, 1985). Long-grain (intermediate-amylose) parboiled rices are preferred in most canning formulations because of the required cooked rice stability. Non-parboiled high-amylose rices, particularly those with a hard gel consistency, are also suitable, but the texture may be too hard. A pH below 4.6 is recommended for canned rice to reduce microbial contamination because retorted canned rice may not be completely sterilized.

In Japan, low-amylose milled rice is placed in cans with water, broth or another seasoning, steamed for about 30 minutes and sealed and sterilized in a retort at 112°C for 80 minutes (Juliano and Sakurai, 1985). Canned rice is heated in boiling water for 15 minutes before serving. Canned seasoned cooked rice is marketed primarily as military rations and as emergency foods. Intermediate-amylose rice is used in canned rice for the military in the Philippines. Annual production of canned rice in Japan was 1 472 t in 1983, but it is declining in popularity (Tani, 1985) with only 1 159 t produced in 1986 (Iwasaki, 1987).

Both wet- and dry-pack canned rices are produced in Taiwan (Chang, 1988). Daily production of wet-pack rice is 360 000 easy-to-open 340-ml cans, while the production of dry-pack rice is very limited. Wet-pack canned rice preparations, usually called rice congee, use waxy rice and are all sweetened; the most popular formula includes waxy rice as a base together with dried longans, red beans, peanuts, oatmeal and sugar. Low-amylose rice is used for dry-pack fried rice.

FERMENTED RICE PRODUCTS

Various waxy rice wines are prepared by fermenting steamed waxy milled rice with fungi and a yeast starter (Steinkraus, 1983; Juliano and Sakurai, 1985). A sweet product is first produced, which is then converted to alcohol as fermentation progresses. The liquid is removed by decantation. Examples are Chinese *lao-chao*, Thai *khaomak*, Malaysian *tapai*, Indonesian *tape ketan* and Philippine *tapuy*. Red rices are preferred for *tapuy* and are often roasted before cooking (Sanchez *et al.*, 1989). Ethanol conversion is higher for waxy and low-amylose rice than for intermediate- and high-amylose rice during *tapuy* production; undigested starch is mainly amylose (Sanchez *et al.*, 1988).

Rice wine production in Taiwan uses 67 000 t of milled rice annually and uses either *Aspergillus oryzae* (*shao-hsing* wine) or *Rhizopus* sp. (*hua-tiao*) for saccharification (Chang, 1988). Overmilled waxy rice (20 percent bran polish) is washed, steeped in water, steamed, inoculated with *A. oryzae* spores and incubated for 45 hours at 35 to 38°C for a low-amylose brown rice starter.

Ragi-type starters (*bubod* in the Philippines) are available in the markets of most Asian countries (Steinkraus, 1983). They are usually small (3 to 6 cm), round, flattened cakes of rice flour on which the desired micro-organisms have been grown. The cakes are either air-dried or sun-dried and the dehydration occurs simultaneously with growth of the organisms. Micro-organisms include the mould *Rhizopus* sp. or combinations of the essential yeasts and moulds required for the different types of alcoholic fermentations.

Rice is the sole cereal substrate in Japanese rice wine such as *sake* (Yoshizawa and Kishi, 1985). The raw material is highly milled rice (25 to 30 percent bran polish by weight of brown rice) with low amylose, low GT and a white core, characteristics that facilitate swelling, cooking and penetration by the mycelia of *A. oryzae*. Overmilling lowers protein (5 to 6 percent) and non-starch lipids (0.1 percent) and also potassium and phosphorus levels. Steamed rice is inoculated with *koji*, a culture of *A. oryzae* grown on steamed rice and seed mash. *Sake* yeast is grown on *koji* steamed rice containing 70 ml lactic acid per 100 litres of water at 12°C.

Three more additions of materials are made to maintain fermentation. About 500 000 t of milled rice were used for *sake* in Japan in 1985 (Tani, 1985).

Rice milk has been used as a substitute for animal milk and milk powder and may be prepared either from puffed rice flour or from wet milled flour with sugar and peanut oil for flavouring. Brown rice gives a better-quality milk than milled rice, and a formulation of 3.5 percent (wt/vol.) of brown rice, 2 percent peanut oil and 7.5 percent sugar gave the best sensory score (Lin, Shao and Chiang, 1988). Rice milk contains 87.7 percent moisture, 0.8 percent protein, 0.8 percent fat, 0.1 percent crude fibre, 0.1 percent ash and 10.4 percent carbohydrate; it has 11 percent total solids and viscosity of <3 poise. Use of bacterial amylases to hydrolyse the starch can increase the solids content of the milk without unduly increasing the milk viscosity (Mitchell, Mitchell and Nissenbaum, 1988).

Mirin is a clear, sweet drink made by adding steamed waxy rice and *koji* to *shochu*, a gin-like alcoholic beverage obtained by distilling a type of *sake* made from broken indica rice. The mixture is allowed to ferment in the presence of 40 percent ethanol from *shochu* until the rice starch is converted to sugars (two months at 25 to 30°C). After filtration and treatment with tannin and gluten and refiltering, the bottled *mirin* contains 14 percent ethanol and 45 percent sugars. It is used either for drinking (sweetened *sake*) or for seasoning Japanese dishes. *Mirin* production in 1986 in Japan was 78 000 kl (Sagara, 1988).

Rice vinegar results from the completion of the rice starch fermentation and is a traditional Japanese and Chinese product (Iwasaki, 1987). Acetic acid fermentation is carried out by mixing seed vinegar with the rice wine and takes one to three months. The product is ripened, filtered, pasteurized and bottled (Lai, Chang and Luh, 1980). It has 4 to 5 percent total acidity (mostly acetic acid, plus some lactic and succinic acids). Rice vinegar production in Japan was 40 000 kl in 1983 (Tani, 1985) and 52 000 kl in 1986 (Sagara, 1988).

Broken rice, together with maize grits, is an adjunct in beer manufacture in the United States and Japan (Yoshizawa and Kishi, 1985). Rice is preferred to maize because of its lower protein and fat content (<1.5 percent). Broken rice is obtained from regular milling of brown rice in most countries, except in Japan, where it is milled from broken brown rice. Broken rice must be free from bran contamination to reduce protein and fat content. Low-GT, low-amylose rices are used because intermediate-GT, intermediate-amylose rices are relatively resistant to starch liquefaction. Rice seed is not used for malting in place of barley because of its lower α-amylose production (IRRI, 1988b).

Other fermented rice products include Japanese *miso*, Sierra rice (*amarillo* or *requemado*) from Latin America and *angkak* (*anka*, red rice). *Miso* is a traditional Japanese brown seasoning paste principally used for a breakfast soup. It is prepared from *koji* (*A. oryzae*) from milled rice mixed with cooked and minced soybean, salt and a starter of cultured yeast and lactic acid bacteria. The ingredients are fermented in covered vats at 25 to 30°C for one to three months (Wang, 1980). The rice-to-soybean ratio is about 2:1. Japanese *miso* production in 1986 was 471 000 kl (Sagara, 1988). Sierra rice is derived from moist rough rice fermented by the micro-organisms that are naturally present with heating up to 50 to 70°C. The grain becomes yellow to brown and is essentially precooked and predigested. *Angkak* may be produced by *Monascus purpureus* mould on cooked rice at 35 percent moisture and pH 6.5 at room temperature (Dizon and Sanchez, 1984). It is used as a colouring agent for food, such as fermented fish (Hesseltine, 1979).

RICE FLOURS AND STARCH
Rice flour in Japan is made from both waxy and non-waxy rices and from both raw and gelatinized rice. It is milled by rolling, pounding, shock-milling, stone-milling, milling in a lateral steel mill and wet milling in a stone mill. In 1985, rice flour production in Japan included 67 000 t from raw rice plus 140 t from pregelatinized rice (Tani, 1985). In 1987, rice flour production used 105 000 t of brown rice (Hirao, 1990).

A tea prepared from roasted brown rice in Japan used 23 800 t of non-waxy and 1 200 t of waxy rice in 1985 (Tani, 1985). Production in 1986 was 20 000 t (Sagara, 1988).

High-protein rice flours for early childhood feeding may be obtained from cooked milled rice by destarching treatment with α-amylase (Resurrección,

Juliano and Eggum, 1978; Hansen *et al.*, 1981). A high-fructose rice syrup and a high-protein rice flour have been produced from broken rice using α-amylase, glucoamylase and glucose isomerase. This procedure obtained an 80 percent glucose yield from brokens (91 percent starch basis) which was converted to 50 percent glucose, 42 percent fructose and 3 percent maltose (Chen and Chang, 1984). The high-protein flour (28 percent protein) was recovered in 30 to 32 percent yield. Others have obtained 80 percent protein flour (Resurrección, Juliano and Eggum, 1978). Malto-dextrins are also produced from milled rice flour at 80°C using heat-stable α-amylase (Griffin and Brooks, 1989).

Rice starch production involves mainly wet milling of brokens with 0.3 to 0.5 percent sodium hydroxide to remove protein (Juliano, 1984). Brokens are steeped in alkali solution for 24 hours and are then wet milled in pin mills, hammermills or stone-mill disintegrators with the alkali solution. After the batter is stored for 10 to 24 hours, fibre (cell wall) is removed by passing it through screens; the starch is collected by centrifugation, washed thoroughly with water and dried. Protein in the effluent may be recovered by neutralization and the precipitated protein used as a feed supplement.

In the European Economic Community (EEC), about 8 800 t of broken rice are processed annually to about 7 000 t of starch in five to six plants in Belgium, Germany, Italy and the Netherlands (Kempf, 1984). The starch is used exclusively as a human food, largely for baby foods and also in extruded noodles. Egypt, Syria and Thailand also produce rice starch.

RICE BRAN AND RICE-BRAN OIL

Rice bran has been an extremely popular source of dietary fibre because of the hypocholesterolaemic property of its oil fraction. Stabilized rice bran has been made available by the use of the Brady extruder in the United States to stabilize the full-fat bran by inactivating its lipase (Saunders, 1990). It is finding application in breakfast cereals, snack foods and bakery products. Stabilized rice bran has been incorporated into whole-wheat bread, muffins, peanut butter cookies and oatmeal cookies at levels of up to 20 percent. The 3 to 8 percent sugar content of rice bran may also contribute to oven browning. The high water absorption capacity of rice bran helps maintain moisture and freshness and therefore improves shelf-life. Its foaming capacity aids in air incorporation and leavening.

In tropical Asia, food applications of rice bran will have to await the reduction of hull contamination of rice bran from the use of Engelberg mills. However, stabilized rice bran is a good poultry feed since its trypsin inhibitor has been inactivated by extrusion cooking.

Rice-bran oil production was about 679 000 t in 1990 (FAO Statistics Division data) or about 13 percent of potential production based on 7 percent bran from rough rice, 15 percent oil recovery from bran and a world rice production of 507 million tonnes. The principal producers of rice bran oil are India (370 000 t), Japan (83 000 t) and China, including Taiwan (122 000 t).

Rice-bran oil has an iodine absorption number of 92 to 115 and contains 29 to 42 percent linoleic acid and 0.8 to 1.0 percent linolenic acid (Jaiswal, 1983). It is considered a salad oil rich in vitamin E and in various plant sterols (Juliano, 1985b).

RICE TYPES PREFERRED FOR RICE PRODUCTS

Most rice products have a preferred amylose type which is related to the preferred rice type for boiled rice consumption in the country (Table 45). All rice types are used for parboiled rice, but usually intermediate- and high-amylose rices are used in Thailand and the United States. High-amylose rices are used in Bangladesh, India, Pakistan and Sri Lanka. Canned, precooked and quick-cooking rices, expanded rice products, rice cereals and snacks are of the type preferred for boiled rice. Low-GT rices are preferred for fermented products since the rice starch can be gelatinized at 70°C and therefore requires less cooling before inoculation. Low-fat or highly milled rice, preferably freshly milled to minimize rancid odours, is preferred for rice products. Waxy rices are preferred for desserts and sweets because of the slower rate of hardening of the boiled or steamed rice starch.

EFFECT OF PROCESSING ON NUTRITIONAL VALUE

Thermal processes can affect protein and starch properties (Table 46). The effect of boiling and parboiling was discussed in Chapter 5. Yellow rice from

TABLE 45

Amylose type and other properties preferred for processed rice products

Product	Amylose type				Other properties
	Waxy	Low	Intermediate	High	
Parboiled rice[a]	+	+	⊕	⊕	
Precooked and quick-cooking rice[a]	+	+	+	+	
Canned rice[a]	+	+	+	+	
Expanded rice products	+	+	+	+	(Amylose content not a major factor)
Rice cereals and snacks	+	+	+		Low fat; texture affected by amylose content
Extrusion-cooked rice foods		+	+	+	Low fat
Rice-based infant formulations		+	+		Low fat
Rice flour and rice starch	+	+	+	+	Wet milling process, freshly milled
Rice puddings and breads		+	+	+	Low GT
Rice cakes	+	+	+		Low GT, aged (for fermented cakes), freshly milled
Flat rice noodles and rice paper		(+)	⊕		
Extruded rice noodles				+	Hard gel consistency
Rice wines	⊕	⊕	+	+	Low protein and fat; higher ethanol yield for waxy and low amylose
Beer adjunct		+			Low GT and low fat
Fermented rice foods (*idli, dosai*)				+	Parboiled
Rice frozen sauces, desserts, sweets	+	+			Slow retrogradation (syneresis)

[a] Preferred amylose type based on type of raw rice preferred.
⊕ Most preferred amylose type.

stack-burning of wet rough rice has a lower lysine content and NPU than normal rice (Eggum *et al.*, 1984). Cystine and tryptophan are not affected. Extrusion cooking reduces lysine and cystine levels but not tryptophan, and reduces the NPU of milled-rice protein (Eggum *et al.*, 1986). Hydrogen sulphide is observed during rice extrusion cooking. Other heat processes

TABLE 46

Effect of heat treatment and processing on the lysine and cystine content and net protein utilization of rice in growing rats

Processing method	Percent decrease in			References
	Lysine	Cystine	NPU	
Boiling, 20 min	1-3	0	0	Eggum, Resurrección & Juliano, 1977
Pressure parboiling (20-60 min, 120°C, 35% H_2O)	0	0	0	Eggum et al., 1984
Noodle extrusion (35% H_2O, 55°C)	0-3	–	–	Khandker et al., 1986
Pan baking (220-230°C, 7-10 min)	0		0	Khan & Eggum, 1978
Accelerated aging (100°C, 3 hours, sealed)	3		–	IRRI, 1984a
Pan toasting	5		–	IRRI, 1984a
Stackburning (high H_2O, <100°C)	9-18		6-12	Eggum et al., 1984
Induced yellowing (60°C, 4 days, sealed) 25-26% H_2O 14% H_2O	14-18 9		– –	IRRI, 1984a IRRI, 1984a
Popping, brown rice (207°C, 45 sec)	16-17		–	IRRI, 1984a
Extrusion cooking, flour (15% H_2O, 150°C, 45 bars)	11	21	7-8	Eggum et al., 1986
Gun-puffing, milled rice (200-210°C)	0	48	–	Villareal & Juliano, 1987
Commercial steaming and puffing, milled rice	37	–	–	IRRI, 1984a
Manufacture of commercial rice krispies	53	–	41	Khan & Eggum, 1979
Roasting (220-280°C, 2-2.5 min)	69	–	61	Chopra & Hira, 1986

decompose lysine (IRRI, 1984a; Juliano, 1985a), except gun-puffing, which affects cysteine (Villareal and Juliano, 1987). The subsequent toasting step is probably where the lysine decomposition occurs (Khan and Eggum, 1979; Chopra and Hira, 1986). The tryptophan residues in model food proteins are more stable during processing and storage than methionine and lysine (Nielsen et al., 1985).

Rice batter (dough) fermentation reduces the phytate content of 0.45 percent by 45 percent after one day, 74 percent after two days and 80 percent after three days (Marfo *et al.*, 1990). Legume phytate hydrolysis is also reported during fermentation of *idli*.

ENRICHMENT AND FORTIFICATION

The purpose of rice enrichment and fortification is to restore to milled rice the levels of B vitamins and minerals removed from the grain during milling. It is technically more difficult than enriching wheat flour since rice is consumed as a whole grain. Traditional methods include parboiling, acid parboiling with 1 percent acetic acid, thiamine enrichment, coating, production of artificial rice, dibenzoyl-thiamine enrichment and multinutrient enrichment by adding a nutrient-enriched premix (Mickus and Luh, 1980; Misaki and Yasumatsu, 1985). Premix is made by soaking milled rice in an acetic acid solution of the water-soluble vitamins thiamine, riboflavin, niacin, pantothenic acid and pyridoxine. Then it is steamed, dried and coated with separate layers of vitamin E, calcium and iron and then with a protective coating material and natural food colouring to prevent the loss of nutrients through washing. The nutrient levels are the same as those of brown rice. This multinutrient-enriched rice is blended with milled rice at a 1:200 ratio. Only 10 percent of any nutrient is lost through ordinary washing before cooking and another 10 percent on cooking.

The pioneering enrichment field studies in Bataan province, the Philippines in 1948-50 demonstrated that rice enrichment was practical, with striking reductions in the incidence of beriberi in the areas in which enrichment was introduced (Salcedo *et al.*, 1950; Williams, 1956).

Obstacles to the successful introduction of rice enrichment by the premix method include the following (FAO, 1954):
- the cost of the imported premix,
- the difficulty of ensuring that the premix is added to milled rice in the correct proportion in the mill,
- the slightly greater cost of enriched rice as compared with that of ordinary rice, which affects its sale to lower income groups,
- losses of added vitamins which may occur when enriched rice is cooked

in excess water that is subsequently discarded, according to current practice in some rice-eating countries,

• issues related to standards and analysis, particularly of imported rice,

• lack of knowledge about the loss of added nutrients during storage.

Undermilling has been employed to retain B vitamins in milled rice, but the shelf-life of undermilled rice is shorter than that of milled rice and the product is less white (FAO, 1954). Some consumers remill the undermilled rice to remove the rancid outer layer and to make the rice whiter, with an accompanying loss of B vitamins. Milled rice has also been used for enrichment programmes for vitamin A as well as vitamin B in Thailand and the Philippines (Gershoff *et al.*, 1977). The results of a village-wide supplementation of lysine, threonine, thiamine, riboflavin and vitamin A for Thai preschool children were not conclusive with respect to the lysine-threonine fortification.

Chapter 7
Challenges and prospects

KEEPING PACE WITH POPULATION GROWTH

The world population of 5 000 million in 1990 is expected to reach 8 000 million by 2020. Populations of less-developed countries, presently totalling 3 700 million, will reach 6 700 million by 2020. The present 2 100 million rice consumers in developing countries will reach 3 700 million in 2020 (IRRI, 1989).

To meet the projected growth in demand for rice (making allowances for its substitution by other foods) as incomes increase, the 1988 rice production of 490 million tonnes must increase to 556 million tonnes by 2000, and to 758 million tonnes by 2020 — a 65 percent increase (1.7 percent per year), (IRRI, 1989). However, for the leading rice-growing countries of South and Southeast Asia, the needed increase in rice production by 2020 is about 100 percent (2.1 percent per year).

ENVIRONMENTAL CONSIDERATIONS

There has been increasing concern over the growth in aggregate rice output, which has peaked and is starting to decline, according to long-term experiments (IRRI, 1990b). Comparison of data from farmers' fields and experiment stations in Indonesia, the Philippines and Thailand confirmed that yield potentials are stagnating and that there is a diminished gap between potential and actual farm yields. There is also strong but not conclusive evidence that rice yields and productivity are declining more than those of wheat in rice-wheat cropping systems. Zinc deficiency and yield response to phosphorus in addition to nitrogen are now more common.

Current production trends address the stability and ecological sustainability of rice production, its economic viability and equity. Thus, organic fertilizers such as *Sesbania* species and biological nitrogen fixation with organisms such as *Azolla* and *Anabaena* species are being pursued as partial substitutes for inorganic N fertilizers. Nitrogen fertilizer efficiency is only about 40 to 50 percent because of ammonia volatilization, nitrification and denitrification, leaching and surface drainage. Losses may be minimized by the use of slow-release and controlled-release fertilizers (De Datta, 1989). Deep placement either by hand or machine has also shown promising possibilities, but tests on machine deep placement have not given consistent results. Optimum time of split application of nitrogen fertilizer needs to be studied further with the current short-duration varieties. A recent review (Conway and Pretty, 1988) suggests that fertilizer use in developing countries presents very little actual hazard to health and contamination of the environment.

Integrated pest management is being introduced to minimize pesticide use and its concomitant pollution problem. The escalating use of insecticides in rice-growing areas from the 1960s to the 1980s was not balanced by widespread improvements in insect pest control (IRRI, 1984b). Undesirable consequences have included pest resurgence, multiple insecticide resistance of major pests in high-use areas, destruction of communities of natural enemies, drastic reduction of fish as a local protein source and disturbing increases in human and farm-animal poisoning. A framework for long-term stable crop protection should be based on the primary control tactics of varietal resistance, cultural control and biological control. When such control tactics fail to provide adequate protection, insecticides may be applied in relation to pest populations and economic damage levels. The banning of persistent use of pesticides in most rice-producing countries has considerably reduced the pesticide residue and pollution problem. For example, carbofuran residues were found to be below the 0.2 ppm tolerance limit in rough rice from rice plants treated with 0.5 to 1.0 kg/ha active ingredient by various methods (Seiber *et al.*, 1978). Levels of total organophosphate pesticides in irrigation water runoff from the IRRI farm in 1987-88 were low (at the ppb level) on the average, and no organochlorine pesticides were detected (IRRI, 1988b).

Environmental problems related to rice production include global climate changes: increases in atmospheric carbon dioxide, methane and nitrous oxide and a decrease in stratospheric ozone with a resultant increase in the ultraviolet-B radiation reaching the earth's surface, retention of solar radiation (the greenhouse effect) and global warming. Rice fields have been cited as the major generators of methane and nitrous oxide; studies are under way to verify these observations (IRRI, 1990a).

Soil loss in the 13 percent upland rice area (18 million ha) is estimated to be 2 to 4 cm per year or the equivalent of 200 to 400 t/ha per year in the open-field agricultural systems in Southeast Asia (IRRI, 1990b). Indicative of this problem is the fact that major rivers in Southeast Asia carry ten times more sediment out to sea than river systems in other parts of the world.

Water-induced land degradation includes waterlogging and salinity development from the intensive use of land in irrigated conditions. In addition, excessive sedimentation from mine tailings and industrial pollution affects land productivity (IRRI, 1990b). Irrigation management for sustainable production systems is imperative, including water management for acid sulphate soils and productivity enhancement for coastal saline areas. For non-irrigated farms, rainwater conservation in a reservoir of about 7 percent of the farm area can help stabilize yield and increase productivity in rain-fed, drought-prone lowland areas.

Malaria, schistosomiasis and Japanese encephalitis are important vector-borne diseases associated with rice production in developing countries (IRRI, 1988a). The causal agents are directly or indirectly associated with aquatic environments. Mosquitoes are the infective agents of malaria and of the encephalitis virus. Snail species act as intermediate hosts for the schistosome parasites, the cercariae, which swim about freely in contaminated water after they have been shed by the snails.

INCREASING YIELD POTENTIAL

More than 60 percent of the world's rice area is now planted to varieties of improved plant type. Little improvement in yield potential has occurred since the introduction of improved varieties in the mid-1960s when efforts were directed toward incorporating disease and insect resistance, shortening growth duration and improving grain quality. Yield is a function of total dry matter and harvest index (panicle/panicle and straw). The semi-dwarf varieties have a harvest index of around 0.45 to 0.50, in contrast to about 0.3

to 0.4 for the traditional tall varieties (Yoshida, 1981). Efforts are being made to improve the harvest index to around 0.6 to increase yields. The modern varieties have 20 to 25 tillers, of which only about 15 to 16 produce small panicles with about 100 to 120 grains. Efforts are being made to breed rice with only four to five productive tillers but with large panicles of about 250 grains to give a maximum yield of 13 t/ha as compared to the maximum yield of 10 t/ha of the present varieties (IRRI, 1989). These rices must have sturdy stems to support large panicles, dark green erect and thick leaves and a vigorous root system, and they should be about 90 cm tall. The proposed plant type will have to be managed differently from the present high-tillering modern rices which have been bred for transplanted conditions. They will be more suitable for direct sowing. The genetic diversification of tropical rice is being increased by crossing with japonica rices and with wild species through wide hybridization.

Drought resistance is important, particularly in upland and rain-fed lowland rices. Factors such as rooting depth, extent of stomatal closure and cuticular resistance to water vapor are involved in varietal differences in response to water stress.

Deep-water or floating rices have a trait that enables their internodes to elongate to keep up with increases in water level. Deep-water conditions prevail in deltas, estuaries and river valleys in Bangladesh, Cambodia,

Direct-seeded irrigated rice plant of the future, together with traditional and semi-dwarf plant types

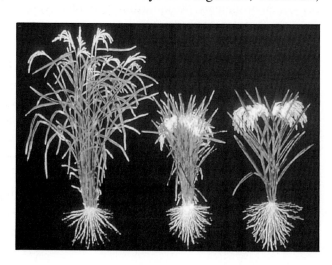

India, Indonesia, Myanmar, Thailand and Viet Nam where flood waters rise annually to depths of from 0.5 to 5 m. Some of these rices also show drought resistance. Cold tolerance at the seedling, tillering or maturity stage is important in the mountains and hilly regions of countries such as Bangladesh, India, Indonesia, Nepal and the Philippines, where the semi-dwarf rices turn yellow and die or are stunted because of low ambient-air or irrigation-water temperatures. However, in the hot regions, such as southern Iran, Pakistan and Senegal, sterility is the problem, mainly because of disturbed pollen shedding and pollen viability.

No modern varieties have been bred to withstand completely the acid sulphate soils in parts of India, Viet Nam, etc.; the salty soils in inland desert areas in parts of India and Pakistan and the salt in brackish water in coastal regions; alkali soils; or organic soils (histosols). Iron toxicity and iron, zinc and phosphorus deficiencies are serious soil problems.

Losses due to insects, diseases and weeds in individual countries in the region range from 10 percent to more than 30 percent. Because of the rapid breakdown of single dominant gene resistance of rice plants to insect pests (about three years for resistance to brown planthopper, the *Bph1* gene), durable moderate resistance is a major focus. This type of resistance is sought to regulate the selection pressure on the insect pests so that insect strains resistant to the rice variety will not readily develop by mutation, genetic drift (the process by which smaller subpopulations hold random subsets of the total genetic variation), migration or selection. More insect population genetic studies are needed to determine how genetic variation in the pests' ability to feed on resistant varieties differs among subpopulations. To manage resistance, we need to understand how both populations and regions differ in genetic variation to overcome resistance. Approaches include pyramiding two or more resistance genes, the multiline approach and horizontal resistance. Wide crosses with wild *Oryza* species are being used to incorporate resistance genes from wild rices. The same strategy is required for all pest resistance genes.

Probably as important a factor as seed viability is seed vigour, which tends to deteriorate during the few months of seed storage after harvest, depending on the variety. Loss of seed vigour results in an uneven initial stand of the rice crop, particularly on direct seeding (Seshu, Krishnasamy and Siddique, 1988). This is particularly critical for direct-seeded irrigated rice, where the pregerminated grain is drilled at least an inch below the soil surface under water. To improve overall productivity not only rice but the whole Asian rice farming system should be considered to determine the best pattern for each region.

RICE BIOTECHNOLOGY

The Rockefeller Foundation's International Programme on Rice Biotechnology, established in 1984, has the following goals: to assure that new techniques for crop genetic improvement based on advances in molecular and cellular biology are developed for rice; to facilitate the transfer of these biotechnologies to rice breeding programmes in the developing world to produce improved varieties that address priority needs; and to help build the scientific research capability necessary for the continued development and application of new rice genetic improvement technologies in selected developing countries (Toenniessen and Herdt, 1989). Activities include wide hybridization to transfer useful traits from wild relatives to cultivated rice and the development of a knowledge base and biotechnology tools. These include the development of genetic maps and markers based on cloned DNA sequences, protoplast techniques as a vehicle for various genetic manipulations, genetic transformation techniques, cloning and characterizing of rice genes, diagnostic tools for the study of host-pathogen interactions and novel genes for rice improvement. Novel genes being studied for rice improvement include viral genes such as a coat-protein gene conferring resistance to rice tungro virus, *Bacillus thuringiensis* toxin genes for resistance to yellow stem borer and other insect pests and wheat genes for inhibitors of rice weevil amylase. The objective is to produce transgenic rice plants containing these useful genes to confer resistance or tolerance to pests and diseases or to environmental stresses in order to ensure stable, high yields.

Efforts are being made to incorporate the maize *Y1* gene (endosperm ß-carotene), (Buckner, Kelson and Robertson, 1990) or a provitamin A carotenoid (e.g. tomato phytonene) gene (Cheung and Kawata, 1990) into rice grain to reduce the incidence of vitamin A deficiency in Asia (see Chapter 2). However, a non-pigmented precursor, as in white as opposed to yellow maize, is preferred to avoid the consumer objection to yellow-endosperm rice. The genes for carotenoid synthesis are present in rice, as in all photosynthetic plants, but are expressed in photosynthetic tissue and not in the endosperm.

Maize and wheat inhibitors of α-amylase from insects, especially the rice weevil, are being examined for possible incorporation into rice grain to improve its shelf-life and reduce storage losses. Oryzacystatin also inhibits rice-weevil digestive enzymes (sulphhydryl protease) and is under study (Reeck, Muthukrishnan and Kramer, 1990).

The wheat glutelin gene involved in bread-baking quality (MacRitchie, du Cros and Wrigley, 1990) is being introduced into rice. The effect of the introduced gene on the grain protein content and quality of transgenic rice plants may be interesting. A wheat high-molecular-weight glutenin gene accumulates in transgenic tobacco endosperm at approximately 0.1 percent of total endosperm protein (Robert, Thompson and Flavell, 1989). Introduction of the barley α-amylose gene may also improve the seed vigour and malting quality of rice grain.

STARCH MUTANTS

Starch mutants from Japanese rices have been induced by treatments of Sasanishiki with ethyl methane sulphonate, of Norin 8 with ^{32}P beta rays, or of fertilized egg cells of Kinmaze with *N*-methyl-*N*-nitrosourea (Omura and Satoh, 1984; Juliano *et al.*, 1990). They have been transferred to IR36 by two back-crosses. *Sugary* mutants contain phytoglycogen and have a high content of free sugars. *Shrunken* mutants have a low starch content. Both *sugary* and *shrunken* mutants have wrinkled brown rice, but the endosperm is hard in *sugary* and soft in *shrunken* mutants (Omura and Satoh, 1984). *Floury* grain has a chalky, soft endosperm. *Dull* mutants contain 2 to 14 percent amylose on a starch basis (as compared to 0 to 2 percent in waxy rice starch) and have a tombstone-white hard endosperm. *Amylose extender* (*ae*) mutants contain irregularly shaped starch granules characteristic of high-amylose maize starch. The IR36-based mutants had lighter, lower-density grains than IR36 and had a higher amylose content than the original Japanese rice mutants except for the *dull* mutants (Juliano *et al.*, 1990).

The IR36-based *ae* mutants have a 40 to 42 percent apparent amylose content and a GT of 73 to 80°C (Juliano *et al.*, 1990). Their protein lysine content is higher than that of IR36 by 0.8 percent in brown rice and 0.5 percent in milled rice (Juliano *et al.*, 1990). The maize *ae* mutant also has a higher lysine content in its protein (Glover *et al.*, 1975). This *ae* mutant and other endosperm starch mutants have SDS-polyacrylamide gel electrophoresis patterns identical to those of the parent varieties (IRRI, 1983b; IRRI, unpublished data, 1990).

PROTEIN MUTANTS

Higher lysine mutants produced by *S*-2-aminoethyl-L-cysteine treatment of United States rices (Schaeffer and Sharpe, 1983) had a higher percentage of lysine in the grain protein (by about 0.5 percent) and a higher percentage of protein in the grain, but they also had lighter grain and actually contained no more lysine than the parent (Juliano, 1985a). The 0.5 percent increase was also reflected in the screening of the rice germplasm bank for lysine content (Juliano, Antonio and Esmama, 1973). *Amylose extender* mutants of IR36 also had 0.5 percent more lysine in their protein than IR36 (Juliano *et al.*, 1990).

A screening programme was initiated for mutants for the rice storage protein bodies PB-I and PB-II, which are located in the starchy endosperm. The crystalline PB-II is rich in glutelin and the large, spherical PB-I is rich in prolamin (see Chapter 3). Glutelin has a better amino acid score than prolamin except for that of a minor subunit of prolamin (see Table 17). Thus, the aim of the screening programme was to improve the nutritional quality of the rice protein by increasing the proportion of PB-II proteins, or reducing the proportion of PB-I proteins (Kumamaru *et al.*, 1988). A number of mutants were identified which met these criteria, and their protein bodies were isolated and characterized (Ogawa *et al.*, 1989).

Rice/sorghum and rice/wheat hybrids from the People's Republic of China were also rechecked for amino acid composition, particularly lysine, because rice protein is richer in lysine (3.5 to 4 percent) than sorghum (1 to 2 percent lysine) and wheat (2 to 3 percent). The lysine content of four milled rice/sorghum hybrids of 3.1 to 3.6 g per 16.8 g N was closer to rice than to sorghum (IRRI, 1980). One milled sample of rice/wheat hybrid had 4.1 g lysine per 16.8 g N at 10.8 percent protein, with an SDS-polyacrylamide gel electrophoresis pattern characteristic of milled rice glutelin (IRRI, 1983a).

Studies on the biosynthesis of storage proteins in developing rice seeds (Yamagata *et al.*, 1982) indicate that a rice glutelin and a soybean glycinin have evolved from a common ancestral gene (Higuchi and Fukazawa, 1987). Molecular biologists are studying protein biosynthesis in order to enhance the biosynthesis of glutelin, and thus to improve the nutritional quality of rice protein. An alternative approach is to suppress the biosynthesis of prolamin polypeptides that are low in lysine (see Table 17), such as the 10-kd prolamin subunit, which is probably involved in the indigestible BP-I of cooked rice.

OTHER MUTANTS

Giant embryo mutants have an embryo two to three times the normal size and an increased brown rice lipid content (4 percent as compared to 2.5 percent), (Omura and Satoh, 1984). Some mutants have a thicker aleurone layer (>50 μm as compared to the normal 30 μm), which is seen as a possible means to increase the lipid content of the rice grain. The large embryo mutant variety Hokkai 269 has 14 percent bran as compared to 7 percent for common rice, but it has a lower oil content in the bran of 18 percent versus 21 to 22 percent for common bran (A. Nagao, personal communication, 1990).

Bibliography

Adair, C.R. 1972. Production and utilization of rice. *In* D.F. Houston, ed. *Rice chemistry and technology*, p. 1-5. St Paul, MN, USA, Am. Assoc. Cereal Chem.

Antonio, A.A. & Juliano, B.O. 1973. Amylose content and puffed volume of parboiled rice. *J. Food Sci.*, 38: 915-916.

Aoe, S., Ohta, F. & Ayano, Y. 1989. Effect of rice bran hemicellulose on the cholesterol metabolism in rats. *Nippon Eiyo Shokuryo Gakkaishi*, 42: 55-61.

Asian Development Bank. 1989. *Key indicators of developing member countries of ADB*, Vol. 20. Manila, ADB. 388 pp.

Autret, M., Perisse, J., Sizaret, F. & Cresta, M. 1968. Protein value of different types of diet in the world: their appropriate supplementation. *Nutr. Newsl.*, 6(4): 1-29.

Ayano, Y., Ohta, F., Watanabe, Y. & Mita, K. 1980. "Dietary fiber" fractions in defatted rice bran and their hypocholesterolemic effect in cholesterol-fed rats. *Eiyo To Shokuryo*, 33: 283-291.

Bandara, J.M.R.S. 1985. Study on the relationship between fermented odour, presence of bran and mould in parboiled rice, and aflatoxin content in Sri Lanka. In *FAO/UNDP Regional Field Workshop on Rice Grading, Inspection and Analysis*, Lahore & Karachi, Pakistan, 11-18 March 1985, p. 218-225. Bangkok, FAO Regional Office for Asia and the Pacific.

Barber, S. 1972. Milled rice and changes during aging. *In* D.F. Houston, ed. *Rice chemistry and technology*, p. 215-263. St Paul, MN, USA, Am. Assoc. Cereal Chem.

Barker, R.X., Herdt, R.W. & Rose, B. 1985. *The rice economy of Asia*. Washington, D.C., Resources for the Future; Manila, IRRI. 324 pp.

Bean, M.M. & Nishita, K.D. 1985. Rice flours for baking. *In* B.O. Juliano, ed. *Rice chemistry and technology*, 2nd ed., p. 539-556. St Paul, MN, USA, Am. Assoc. Cereal Chem.

Bechtel, D.B. & Pomeranz, Y. 1978. Ultrastructure of the mature ungerminated rice (*Oryza sativa*) caryopsis. The starchy endosperm. *Am. J. Bot.*, 65: 684-691.

Bhattacharya, K.R. 1985. Parboiling of rice. *In* B.O. Juliano, ed. *Rice chemistry and technology*, 2nd ed, p. 289-348. St Paul, MN, USA, Am. Assoc. Cereal Chem.

Bibby, B.G. 1985. Cereal foods and dental caries. *Cereal Foods World*, 30: 851-855.

Björck, I., Nyman, N., Pedersen, B., Siljeström, M., Asp, N.-G. & Eggum, B.O. 1987. Formation of enzyme resistant starch during autoclaving of wheat starch: studies *in vitro* and *in vivo*. *J. Cereal Sci.*, 6: 159-172.

Blackwell, R.Q., Yang, T.H. & Juliano, B.O. 1966. Effect of protein content upon growth rates of rats fed high-rice diets (Abstr.) *Proc. 11th Pac. Sci. Congr., Tokyo,* 8: 15.

Bradbury, J.H. & Holloway, W.D. 1988. *Chemistry of tropical root crops: significance for nutrition and agriculture in the Pacific.* Canberra, Australian Centre for International Agricultural Research. 201 pp.

Breckenridge, C. & Arseculeratne, S.N. 1986. Laboratory studies on parboiled and raw rough rice and their milling fractions as substrates for the production and accumulation of aflatoxin. *Food Microbiol.*, 3: 67-72.

Bressani, R., Elias, L.G. & Juliano, B.O. 1971. Evaluation of the protein quality of milled rices differing in protein content. *J. Agric. Food Chem.*, 19: 1028-1034.

Brockington, S.F. & Kelly, V.J. 1972. Rice breakfast cereals and infant foods. *In* D.F. Houston, ed. *Rice chemistry and technology*, p. 410-418. St Paul, MN, USA, Am. Assoc. Cereal Chem.

Buckner, B., Kelson, T.L. & Robertson, D.S. 1990. Cloning of the Y_1 locus of maize, a gene involved in the biosynthesis of carotenoids. *Plant Cell*, 2: 867-876.

Burns, E.E. & Gerdes, D.L. 1985. Canned rice foods. *In* B.O. Juliano, ed. *Rice chemistry and technology*, 2nd ed., p. 557-567. St Paul, MN, USA, Am. Assoc. Cereal Chem.

Buttery, R.G., Ling, L.C., Juliano, B.O. & Turnbaugh, J.G. 1983. Cooked rice aroma and 2-acetyl-1-pyrroline. *J. Agric. Food Chem.*, 31: 823-826.

Cabrera, M.I.Z., Loyola, A.S., Alejandro, E.R., Yu, G.B., Kuizon, M.D., Intengan, C. Ll., Roxas, B.V. & Juliano, B.O. 1987. Effect of reduction in energy intake on nitrogen balance and growth of preschool children: a preliminary study. *Philipp. J. Nutr.*, 40: 22-31.

Cabrera-Santiago, M.I., Intengan, C.Ll., Roxas, B.V., Juliano, B.O., Perez, C.M., Loyola, A.S., Alejandro, E.R., Abadilla, J.W., Yu, G.F.B. & Mallillin, A.C. 1986. Protein requirements of preschool children consuming rice-milk, rice-toasted mung bean, and rice diets. *Qual. Plant. Plant Foods Hum. Nutr.*, 36: 167-178.

Cagampang, G.B., Cruz, L.J., Espiritu, S.G., Santiago, R.G. & Juliano, B.O. 1966. Studies on the extraction and composition of rice proteins. *Cereal Chem.*, 43: 145-155.

Cagampang, G.B., Perez, C.M. & Juliano, B.O. 1973. A gel consistency test for eating quality of rice. *J. Sci. Food Agric.*, 24: 1589-1594.

Chang, P.Y. 1988. The utilization of rice in Taiwan, Republic of China. *Food Fert. Technol. Cent. Asian Pac. Reg. Ext. Bull.*, 273: 1-9.

Chang, T.T. 1983. The origins and early cultures of the cereal grains and food legumes. *In* D.N. Keightley, ed. *The origins of Chinese civilization*, p. 65-94. Berkeley, CA, USA, University of California Press.

Chang, T.T. 1985. Crop history and genetic conservation — rice: a case study. *Iowa State J. Res.*, 59: 425-455.

Cheigh, H.-S., Ryu, C.-H., Jo, J.-S. & Kwon, T.-W. 1977a. Effect of washing on the loss of nutrients of rice. *Korean J. Food Sci. Technol.*, 9: 170-174 (in Korean).

Cheigh, H.-S., Ryu, C.-H., Jo, J.-S. & Kwon, T.-W. 1977b. A type of post-harvest loss: nutritional losses during washing and cooking of rice. *Korean J. Food Sci. Technol.*, 9: 229-233.

Chelliah, S. & Heinrichs, E.A. 1984. Factors contributing to rice brown planthopper resurgence. In *Proceedings, FAO/IRRI Workshop on Judicious and Efficient Use of Insecticides on Rice,* IRRI, 21-23 February 1983, p. 107-115. Manila, IRRI.

Chen, W.-P. & Chang, Y.-C. 1984. Production of high-fructose rice syrup and high-protein rice flour from broken rice. *J. Sci. Food Agric.*, 35: 1128-1135.

Chen, X.C., Yin, T.A., Yang, X.J., Bai, J.G. & Huang, Z.S. 1984. Protein requirements of Chinese male adults. *UN Univ. Food Nutr. Bull. Suppl.*, 10: 96-101.

Cheung, A.Y. & Kawata, E. 1990. Isolation of genes involved in carotenoid biosynthesis and accumulation in plants. *Abstracts 4th Annual Meeting Rockefeller Foundation's International Program on Rice Bio-*

technology, IRRI, 9-12 May 1990. New York, Rockefeller Foundation.

Chinnaswamy, R. & Bhattacharya, K.R. 1984. Relationship between amylose content and expansion characteristics of parboiled rice. *J. Cereal Sci.*, 21: 273-279.

Chong, Y.H. 1979. Malnutrition, food patterns and nutritional requirements in Southeast Asia. In *Proceedings UNU/IRRI Workshop on Interfaces Between Agriculture, Nutrition and Food Science*, IRRI, 1977, p. 1-17. Los Baños, Laguna, the Philippines, IRRI.

Chopra, N. & Hira, C.K. 1986. Effect of roasting on protein quality of cereals. *J. Food Sci. Technol.*, 23: 233-235.

Chopra, R.N. 1933. *Indigenous drugs of India*. Calcutta. 655 pp. *Cited in* E. Quisumbing, 1978. *Medicinal plants in the Philippines*. Quezon City, the Philippines, Katha Publishers.

Choudhury, N.H. & Juliano, B.O. 1980. Effect of amylose content on the lipids of mature rice grain. *Phytochemistry*, 19: 1385-1389.

Clark, H.E., Howe, J. M. & Lee, C.J. 1971. Nitrogen retention of adult human subjects fed a high protein rice. *Am. J. Clin. Nutr.*, 24: 324-328.

Clarke, P.A. 1982. Cooking losses in rice — a preliminary study of the effect of grain breakage. *J. Food Technol.*, 17: 507-511.

Codex Alimentarius Commission. 1990. *Proposed draft standard for rice*. FAO Food Standards Programme CX/CPL/90/5. Rome, FAO. 8 pp.

Coffman, W.R. & Juliano, B.O. 1987. Rice. *In* R.A. Olson, ed. *Nutritional quality of cereal grains: genetic and agronomic improvement*. Agron. Monogr. 28, p. 101-131. Madison, WI, USA, American Society of Agronomy/Crop Science Society of America/Soil Science Society of America.

Cogburn, R. R. 1985. Rough rice storage. *In* B.O. Juliano, ed. *Rice chemistry and technology*, 2nd ed., p. 265-287. St Paul, MN, USA, Am. Assoc. Cereal Chem.

Conway, G.R. & Pretty, J.N. 1988. *Fertiliser risks in the developing countries: a review*. London, International Institute for Environment and Development, Sustainable Agriculture Programme. 70 pp.

Dalrymple, D.G. 1986. *Development and spread of high-yielding rice varieties in developing countries*. Washington, D.C., Agency for International Development, Bureau of Science and Technology. 117 pp.

Dans, A.L., Florete, O.G., Paz, E.T., Tamesis, B.R., Añonuevo, J.E. & Zarcilla, F. 1987. The efficacy, safety, and acceptability of high-fiber rice-bran diet (*darak*) in the control of diabetes mellitus. *4th Congress ASEAN Federation of Endocrine Societies*, Manila, 5-10 December.

De Datta, S.K. 1981. *Principles and practices of rice production.* New York, J. Wiley & Sons. 618 pp.

De Datta, S.K. 1989. Integrated nutrient management in relation to soil fertility in lowland rice-based cropping systems. In *Rice farming systems: new directions*, p. 141-160. Manila, IRRI.

del Rosario, A.R., Briones, V.P., Vidal, A.J. & Juliano, B.O. 1968. Composition and endosperm structure of developing and mature rice kernel. *Cereal Chem.*, 45: 225-235.

DeMaeyer, E.M. 1986. Xerophthalmia and blindness of nutritional origin in the Third World. *Child. Trop.*, No. 165.

DeMaeyer, E.M. & Adiels-Tegman, M. 1985. The prevalence of anaemia in the world. *World Health Stat. Q.*, 38(3): 302-316.

de Padua, D. B. 1979. A critical review of the losses in the rice post-production system in some South-east Asian countries. In *Interfaces between agriculture, nutrition, and food science. Proceedings of a UNU-IRRI workshop*, IRRI, 1977, p. 89-104. Los Baños, Laguna, the Philippines, IRRI.

de Padua, D. 1988. Some imperatives in crop drying research. In *Research and development issues in grain postharvest problems in Asia*, p. 31-37. Eschborn, Germany, GTZ Group for Assistance on Systems Relating to Grain after Harvest.

De Vizia, B., Ciccimarra, F., De Cicco, N. & Auricchio, S. 1975. Digestibility of starches in infants and children. *J. Pediatr.*, 86: 50-55.

Desikachar, H.S.R., Raghavandra Rao, S.N. & Ananthachar, T.K. 1965. Effect of degree of milling on water absorption of rice during cooking. *J. Food Sci. Technol.*, 2: 110-112.

Dien, L.D., Trinh, N.B., Lieu, L.T. & Hieu, L.H. 1987. Influence of seasons on several biochemical criteria of rice seeds (*Oryza sativa* L.). *Tap Chi Sinh Hoc*, 9(2): 15-21, 31.

Dizon, E.L. & Sanchez, P.C. 1984. Mass production of red mold rice ("angkak") and stability of the Monascus pigment. *Philipp. Agric.*, 67: 25-41.

Duncan, D.B. 1955. Multiple range

and multiple *F* tests. *Biometrics*, 11: 1-42.

Efferson, J.N. 1985. Rice quality in world markets. In *Rice grain quality and marketing*, p. 1-13. Manila, IRRI.

Eggum, B.O. 1969. Evaluation of protein quality and the development of screening techniques. In *New approaches to breeding for improved plant protein*, p. 125-135. Vienna, IAEA.

Eggum, B.O. 1973. *A study of certain factors influencing protein utilization in rats and pigs.* Publ. 406. Copenhagen, Agricultural Research Laboratory. 173 pp.

Eggum, B.O. 1977. Nutritional aspects of cereal protein. *In* A. Muhammad, R. Aksel & R.C. von Boustel, eds. *Genetic diversity in plants*, p. 349-369. New York, Plenum Press.

Eggum, B.O. 1979. The nutritional value of rice in comparison with other cereals. In *Proceedings, Workshop on Chemical Aspects of Rice Grain Quality*, p. 91-111. Los Baños, Laguna, the Philippines, IRRI.

Eggum, B.O., Alabata, E.P. & Juliano, B.O. 1981. Protein utilization of pigmented and nonpigmented brown and milled rice by rats. *Qual. Plant. Plant Foods Hum. Nutr.*, 31: 175-179.

Eggum, B.O., Cabrera, M.I.Z. & Juliano, B.O. 1992. Protein and lysine digestibility and protein quality of cooked Filipino rice diets and milled rice in growing rats. *Plant Foods Hum. Nutr.*, 42: (in press).

Eggum, B.O. & Juliano, B.O. 1973. Nitrogen balance in rats fed rices differing in protein content. *J. Sci. Food. Agric.*, 24: 921-927.

Eggum, B.O. & Juliano, B.O. 1975. Higher protein content from nitrogen fertilizer application and nutritive value of milled rice protein. *J. Sci. Food Agric.*, 26: 425-427.

Eggum, B.O., Juliano, B.O., Ibabao, M.G.B. & Perez, C.M. 1986. Effect of extrusion cooking on nutritional value of rice flour. *Food Chem.*, 19: 235-240.

Eggum, B.O., Juliano, B.O., Ibabao, M.G.B., Perez, C.M. & Carangal, V.R. 1987. Protein and energy utilization of boiled rice-legume diets and boiled cereals in growing rats. *Qual. Plant. Plant Foods Hum. Nutr.*, 37: 237-245.

Eggum, B.O., Juliano, B.O. & Maniñgat, C.C. 1982. Protein and energy utilization of rice milling fractions by rats. *Qual. Plant. Plant Foods Hum. Nutr.*, 31: 371-376.

Eggum, B.O., Juliano, B.O., Villareal, C.P. & Perez, C.M. 1984.

Effect of treatment on composition and protein and energy utilization of rice and mung bean by rats. *Qual. Plant. Plant Foods Hum. Nutr.*, 34: 261-272.

Eggum, B.O., Resurrección, A.P. & Juliano, B.O. 1977. Effect of cooking on nutritional value of milled rice in rats. *Nutr. Rep. Int.*, 16: 649-655.

El Bayâ, A.W., Nierle, W. & Wolff, J. 1980. Substanzverluste beim Kochen von Reis. *Getreide Mehl Brot*, 34: 43-46.

El-Harith, A.E.-H., Dickerson, J.W.T. & Walker, R. 1976. On the nutritive value of various starches for the albino rat. *J. Sci. Food Agric.*, 27: 521-526.

Ellis, J. R., Villareal, C.P. & Juliano, B.O. 1986. Protein content, distribution and retention during milling of brown rice. *Qual. Plant. Plant Foods Hum. Nutr.*, 36: 17-26.

Englyst, H.N., Anderson, V. & Cummings, J.H. 1983. Starch and non-starch polysaccharides in some cereal foods. *J. Sci. Food Agric.*, 34: 1434-1440.

Eppendorfer, W.H., Eggum, B.O. & Bille, S.W. 1979. Nutritive value of potato crude protein as influenced by manuring and amino acid. *J. Sci. Food Agric.*, 30: 361-368.

FAO. 1954. *Rice and rice diets — a nutritional survey*, rev. ed. Rome, FAO. 78 pp.

FAO. 1984. *Food balance sheets, 1979-81 average*. Rome, FAO.

FAO. 1985. *Rice processing industries. FAO/UNDP Regional Workshop*, Jakarta, 15-20 July 1985. Bangkok, FAO Regional Office for Asia and the Pacific. 293 pp.

FAO. 1990a. Rice. *FAO Q. Bull. Stat.*, 3(1): 20-28, 55, 73.

FAO. 1990b. *FAO production yearbook, 1989*. FAO Stat. Ser. No. 88, Vol. 43. Rome, FAO.

FAO. 1990c. *Protein quality evaluation. Report of a Joint FAO/WHO Expert Consultation*, Bethesda, MD, USA, 4-8 December 1989. Rome, FAO. 66 pp.

FAO. 1991. *Cost of producing rice in selected countries*. FAO Committee on Commodity Problems, Intergovernmental Group on Rice, 34th Session, 25-28 March 1991. Rome, FAO. 37 pp.

Feldstein, H.S. & Poats, S.V. 1990. *Women in rice farming systems review report*. Manila, IRRI. 26+ pp.

Ferretti, R.J. & Levander, O.A. 1974. Effect of milling and processing on the selenium content of grains and cereal products. *J. Agric. Food Chem.*, 22: 1049-1051.

Flinn, J.C. & Unnevehr, L.J. 1984. Contributions of modern rice varieties to nutrition in Asia — an IRRI perspective. *In* P. Pinstrup-Andersen, A. Berg & M. Forman, eds. *International agricultural research and human nutrition*, p. 157-178. Washington, D.C., International Food Policy Research Institute; Rome, UN Administrative Committee on Co-ordination/Subcommittee on Nutrition.

Food and Nutrition Research Institute. 1980. *Food composition tables, recommended for use in the Philippines.* FNRI Handbook 1, 5th rev. Manila, FNRI. 313 pp.

Food and Nutrition Research Institute. 1984. *Second nationwide nutrition survey, Philippines, 1982.* FNRI-84-RP-ns-10. Manila, FNRI. 228 pp.

Food and Nutrition Research Institute, 1987. *Aflatoxin content of selected Filipino food items.* Manila, FNRI, Biological Hazards Section, Food Composition and Quality Program (Unpublished typescript).

Furugori, K. 1985. Rice processing manufacturing industries in Japan. Recent trends in technologies. In *FAO/UNDP Regional Workshop on Rice Processing Industries*, Jakarta, 15-20 July 1985, p. 82-87. Bangkok, FAO Regional Office for Asia and the Pacific.

Gariboldi, F. 1984. *Rice parboiling.* FAO Agric. Serv. Bull. 56. Rome, FAO. 73 pp.

Gerhardt, A.L. & Gallo, N.B. 1989. *Effect of a processed California medium grain rice bran and germ product on hypercholesterolemia.* Poster paper presented at the Annual Meeting, Am. Assoc. Cereal Chem., Washington, D.C.

Gershoff, S.N., McGandy, R.B., Suttapreyasri, D., Promkutkao, C., Nondasuta, A., Pisolyabutra, U., Tantiwongse, P. & Viravaidhyaya, V. 1977. Nutrition studies in Thailand. II. Effect of fortification of rice with lysine, threonine, thiamine, riboflavin, vitamin A and iron on preschool children. *Am. J. Clin. Nutr.*, 30: 1185-1195.

Glover, D.V., Crane, P.L., Misra, P.S. & Mertz, E.T. 1975. Genetics of endosperm mutants in maize as related to protein quality and quantity. In *High quality protein maize, CIMMYT-Purdue University International Symposium,* El Batan, 1972, p. 228-240. Stroudsburg, PA, USA, Dowden, Hutchinson & Ross.

Goddard, M.S., Young, G. & Marcus, R. 1984. The effect of amylose content on insulin and glucose response to ingested rice. *Am. J. Clin. Nutr.*, 39: 388-392.

Gopala Krishna, A.G., Prabhakar, J.V. & Sen, D.P. 1984. Effect of degree of milling on tocopherol content of rice bran. *J. Food Sci. Technol.*, 21: 222-224.

Graham, G.G., Glover, D.V., Lopez de Romaña, G., Morales, E. & MacLean, W.C. Jr. 1980. Nutritional value of normal, opaque-2 and sugary-2 opaque-2 maize hybrids for infants and children. I. Digestibility and utilization. *J. Nutr.*, 110: 1061-1069.

Grewal, P. & Sangha, J.K. 1990. Effect of processing on thiamin and riboflavin contents of some high-yielding rice varieties of Punjab. *J. Sci. Food Agric.*, 52: 387-391.

Griffin, V.K. & Brooks, J.R. 1989. Production and size distribution of rice maltodextrins hydrolyzed from milled rice flour using heat-stable alpha-amylase. *J. Food Sci.*, 54: 190-193.

Habito, C.F. 1987. A stochastic evaluation of mechanized rice post-harvest technology through systems simulation modelling (will reduced risk and uncertainty sell paddy dryers?). *In* B.M. de Mesa, ed. *Grain production in postharvest systems. Proceedings 9th ASEAN Technical Seminar on Grain Postharvest Technology*, Singapore, 26-29 August 1986, p. 253-271. Manila, ASEAN Crops Postharvest Programme.

Hallberg, L., Bjorn-Rasmussen, E., Rossander, L. & Suwanik, R. 1977. Iron absorption from Southeast Asia diets. II. Role of various factors that might explain low absorption. *Am. J. Clin. Nutr.*, 30: 539-548.

Hansen, L.P., Hosek, R., Callon, M. & Jones, F.T. 1981. The development of high protein rice flour for early childhood feeding. *Food Technol.*, 35(1): 38-42.

Haumann, B.F. 1989. Rice bran linked to lower cholesterol. *J. Am. Oil Chem. Soc.*, 66: 615-618.

Hayakawa, T. & Igaue, I. 1979. Studies on the washing of milled rice: scanning electron microscopic observation and chemical study of solubilized materials. *Nippon Nogei Kagaku Kaishi,* 53: 321-327.

Hegsted, D.M. & Juliano, B.O. 1974. Difficulties in assessing the nutritional quality of rice protein. *J. Nutr.*, 104: 772-781.

Hemavathy, J. & Prabhakar, J.V. 1987. Lipid composition of rice (*Oryza sativa* L.) bran. *J. Am. Oil Chem. Soc.*, 64: 1016-1019.

Herdt, R.W. 1986. The economics of rice production in developing countries. *Food Rev. Int.*, 1: 447-463.

Hesseltine, C.W. 1979. Some important fermented foods of mid Asia, the Middle East, and Africa. *J. Am. Oil Chem. Soc.*, 56: 367-374.

Hibino, K., Kidzu, T., Masumura, T., Ohtsuki, K., Tanaka, K., Kawabata, K. & Fujii, S. 1989. Amino acid composition of rice prolamin polypeptides. *Agric. Biol. Chem.*, 53: 513-518.

Higuchi, W. & Fukazawa, C. 1987. A rice glutelin and a soybean glycinin have evolved from a common ancestral gene. *Gene*, 55: 245-253.

Hinton, J.J.C. & Shaw, B. 1954. The distribution of nicotinic acid in the rice grain. *Br. J. Nutr.*, 8: 65-71.

Hirao, M. 1990. Trend of rice consumption in Japan. *Farming Jpn.*, 24(1): 14-20.

Hizukuri, S., Takeda, Y., Maruta, N. & Juliano, B.O. 1989. Molecular structures of rice starch. *Carbohydr. Res.*, 189: 227-235.

Holland, B., Unwin, I.D. & Buss, D.H. 1988. *Cereal and cereal products.* Third Supplement to McCance, R.A. & Widdowson, E.M. *The composition of food*, 4th ed. Nottingham, Royal Society of Chemistry. 147 pp.

Holm, J., Björck, I., Ostrowska, S., Eliasson, A.-C., Asp, N.-G., Larsson, K. & Lundquist, I. 1983. Digestibility of amylose-lipid complexes *in-vitro* and *in-vivo*. *Starch*, 35: 294-297.

Hopkins, D.T. 1981. Effect of variation in protein digestibility. *In* C.E. Bodwell, J.S. Adkins & D.T. Hopkins, eds. *Protein quality in humans: assessment and in vitro estimation*, p. 169-193. Westport, CT, USA, AVI Publishing Co.

Huang, J., David, C.C. & Duff, B. 1991. Rice in Asia: is it becoming an inferior good? (Comment.) *Am. J. Agric. Econ.*, 73: 515-521.

Huang, J.-F. 1990. The relation between soil nutrients and rice qualities. *Trans. 14th Int. Congr. Soil Sci.*, Kyoto, 12-18 Aug. 1990, 4: 170-175.

Huang, P.C. 1987. Changing pattern of rice grain production, consumption and dietary life in Taiwan. In *Proceedings, International Symposium, Dietary Life of Rice-Eating Populations*, Kyoto, 24 October 1987, p. 47-52. Kyoto, Research Institute for Production Development.

Huang, P.C. & Lin, C.P. 1982. Protein requirements of young Chinese male adults on ordinary Chinese mixed diet and egg diet at ordinary levels of energy intake. *J. Nutr.*, 112: 897-907.

Huang, P.C., Lin, C.P. & Hsu, J.Y.

1980. Protein requirements of normal infants at the age of about one year: maintenance nitrogen requirements and obligatory nitrogen losses. *J. Nutr.*, 110: 1727-1735.

Huebner, F.R., Bietz, J.A., Webb, B.D. & Juliano, B.O. 1990. Rice cultivar identification by high-performance liquid chromatography of endosperm proteins. *Cereal Chem.*, 67: 129-135.

Huke, R.E. & Huke, E.H. 1990. *Rice: then and now*. Manila, International Rice Research Institute. 44 pp.

Hussain, T., Tontisirin, K. & Chaowanakarnkit, L. 1983. Protein digestibility of weaning foods prepared from rice-minced meat and rice-mungbean combination in infants using a short term nitrogen balance method. *J. Nutr. Sci. Vitaminol.*, 29: 497-508.

Ilag, L.L. & Juliano, B.O. 1982. Colonisation and aflatoxin formation by *Aspergillus* spp. on brown rices differing in endosperm properties. *J. Sci. Food Agric.*, 33: 97-102.

Imai, T. 1990. Rice-based products in Japan. *Farming Jpn.*, 24(1): 21-28.

Inoue, G., Kishi, K., Fujita, Y., Yamamoto, S. & Yoshimura, Y. 1981. Interrelationships between effects of protein and energy intakes on nitrogen utilization in adult men.

UN Univ. Food Nutr. Bull. Suppl., 5: 247-258.

Intengan, C.Ll., Roxas, B.V., Bautista, C.A. & Alejo, L.G. 1976. Studies on protein requirements of Filipinos. *Philipp. J. Nutr.*, 29: 94-98.

Intengan, C.Ll., Roxas, B.V., Cabrera-Santiago, M.I.Z., Loyola, A.S., Alejandro, E.R., Abadilla, J.N. & Yu, G.F.B. 1984. Protein requirements of Filipino children 18-30 months old concerning local diets. I. Rice-fish and rice-mungbean diets. *Philipp. J. Nutr.*, 37: 87-95.

Intengan, C.Ll., Roxas, B.V., Santiago, M.I. & Juliano, B.O. 1982. Protein requirements of adult Filipinos concerning local diets. *Philipp. J. Nutr.*, 35: 112-119.

IRRI. 1975. *Annual report for 1974*, p. 1-50. Manila, IRRI.

IRRI. 1976. *Annual report for 1975*, p. 83-90, 111-125. Manila, IRRI.

IRRI. 1980. *Annual report for 1979*, p. 25-38. Manila, IRRI.

IRRI. 1983a. *Annual report for 1981*, p. 77-82. Manila, IRRI.

IRRI. 1983b. *Annual report for 1982*, p. 70-75. Manila, IRRI.

IRRI. 1984a. *Annual report for 1983*, p. 61-66. Manila, IRRI.

IRRI. 1984b. *Proceedings of the FAO/*

IRRI Workshop on Judicious and Efficient Use of Insecticides on Rice. Manila, IRRI. 180 pp.

IRRI. 1988a. *Vector-borne disease control in humans through rice agroecosystem management*. Manila, IRRI (in collaboration with WHO/FAO/UNEP Panel of Experts on Environmental Management for Vector Control). 237 pp.

IRRI. 1988b. *Annual report for 1987*, p. 43-54, 188-193. Manila, IRRI.

IRRI. 1989. *IRRI toward 2000 and beyond*. Manila, IRRI. 66 pp.

IRRI. 1990a. *Program report for 1989*, p. 200-205. Manila, IRRI.

IRRI. 1990b. *Sustainability aspects of rice culture*. External review, summary papers. Manila, IRRI.

IRRI. 1991a. *World rice statistics, 1990*. Manila, IRRI. 320 p.

IRRI. 1991b. *Program report for 1990*. Manila, IRRI.

IRRI & IDRC (International Development Research Centre). 1992. *Consumer demand for rice grain quality*. Manila, IRRI (in press).

Iwasaki, T. 1987. *Measures for the enhancement of rice consumption and diversification of rice utilization*. Paper presented at the International Seminar on the Diversification of Rice Utilization, 12-17 October, Bangkok. 3 pp.

Jaiswal, P.K. 1983. Specification of rice bran oil and extractions. In *Rice bran oil: status and prospects. Proceedings of a seminar*, Southern Zone, Hyderabad, 13 August 1983, p. 64-77. Andra Pradesh, Oil Technologists' Association of India.

Jiraratsatit, J., Mangklabruks, A., Keoplung, M., Matayabun, S. & Chumsilp, L. 1987. Glycemic effects of rice and glutinous rice on treated-type II diabetic subjects. *J. Med. Assoc. Thailand*, 70: 401-409.

Juliano, B.O. 1972. The rice caryopsis and its composition. *In* D.F. Houston, ed. *Rice chemistry and technology*, p. 16-74. St Paul, MN, USA, Am. Assoc. Cereal Chem.

Juliano, B.O. 1979. The chemical basis of rice grain quality. In *Proceedings, Workshop on Chemical Aspects of Rice Grain Quality*, p. 69-90. Los Baños, Laguna, the Philippines, IRRI.

Juliano, B.O. 1984. Rice starch: production, properties, and uses. *In* R.L. Whistler, J.N. BeMiller & E.F. Paschall, eds. *Starch: chemistry and technology*, 2nd ed., p. 507-528. Orlando, FL, USA, Academic Press.

Juliano, B.O. 1985a. Factors affecting nutritional properties of rice protein. *Trans. Natl. Acad. Sci. Technol. (Philipp.)*, 7: 205-216.

Juliano, B.O., ed. 1985b. *Rice: chemistry and technology*, 2nd ed. St Paul, MN, USA, Am. Assoc. Cereal Chem. 774 pp.

Juliano, B.O., Antonio, A.A. & Esmama, B.V. 1973. Effects of protein content on the distribution and properties of rice protein. *J. Sci. Food Agric.*, 24: 295-306.

Juliano, B.O. & Bechtel, D.B. 1985. The rice grain and its gross composition. *In* B.O. Juliano, ed. *Rice chemistry and technology*, 2nd ed., p. 17-57. St Paul, MN, USA, Am. Assoc. Cereal Chem.

Juliano, B.O. & Boulter, D. 1976. Extraction and composition of rice endosperm glutelin. *Phytochemistry*, 15: 1601-1606.

Juliano, B.O. & Duff, B. 1989. *Setting priorities for rice grain quality research*. Paper presented at 12th ASEAN Technical Seminar on Grain Postharvest Technology, Surabaya, Indonesia, 29-31 August.

Juliano, B.O. & Duff, B. 1991. Rice grain quality as an emerging research priority in national rice breeding programs. In *Rice grain marketing and quality issues*, p. 55-64. Manila, IRRI.

Juliano, B.O. & Goddard, M.S. 1986. Cause of varietal difference in insulin and glucose responses to ingested rice. *Qual. Plant. Plant Foods Hum. Nutr.*, 36: 35-41.

Juliano, B.O. & Hicks, P.A. 1993. Utilization of rice functional properties to produce rice food products with modern processing technologies. *Int. Rice Comm. Newsl.* (Special Issue: Proc. 17th Session Intl. Rice Comm., 1990), 39: 163-179.

Juliano, B.O., Ibabao, M.G.B., Perez, C.M., Clark, R.B., Maranville, J.W., Mamaril, C.P., Choudhury, N.H., Momuat, C.J.S. & Corpuz, I.T. 1987. Effect of soil sulfur deficiency on sulfur amino acids and elements in brown rice. *Cereal Chem.*, 64: 27-30.

Juliano, B.O., Perez, C.M. & Kaosaard, M. 1990. Grain quality characteristics of export rices in selected markets. *Cereal Chem.*, 67: 192-197.

Juliano, B.O., Perez, C.M., Kaushik, R. & Khush, G.S. 1990. Some grain properties of IR36-based starch mutants. *Starch*, 42: 256-260.

Juliano, B.O., Perez, C.M., Komindr, S. & Banphotkasem, S. 1989a. Properties of Thai cooked rice and noodles differing in glycemic index in noninsulin-dependent diabetics. *Plant Foods Hum. Nutr.*, 39: 369-374.

Juliano, B.O., Perez, C.M., Maranan, C.L., Abansi, C.L. & Duff, B.

1989b. Grain quality characteristics of rice in Philippine retail markets. *Philipp. Agric.*, 72: 113-122.

Juliano, B.O. & Sakurai, J. 1985. Miscellaneous rice products. *In* B.O. Juliano, ed. *Rice chemistry and technology*, 2nd ed., p. 569-618. St Paul, MN, USA, Am. Assoc. Cereal Chem.

Juliano, B.O. & Villareal, C.P. 1991. *Grain characteristics of milled rices grown in rice-producing countries.* Manila, IRRI.

Kagawa, H., Hirano, H. & Kikuchi, F. 1988. Variation in glutelin seed storage protein in rice (*Oryza sativa* L.). *Jpn. J. Breeding*, 38: 327-332.

Kahlon, T.S., Saunders, R.M., Chow, F.I., Chui, M.C. & Betschart, A.A. 1990. Influence of rice bran, oat bran and wheat bran on cholesterol and triglyceride in hamsters. *Cereal Chem.*, 67: 439-443.

Kaosa-ard, M.S. & Juliano, B.O. 1989. *Assessing quality characteristics and price of rice in selected international markets.* Paper presented at 12th ASEAN Technical Seminar on Grain Postharvest Technology, Surabaya, Indonesia, 29-31 August.

Kempf, W. 1984. Recent trends in European Community and West German starch industries. *Starch*, 36: 333-341.

Kennedy, B.M. & Schelstraete, M. 1975. A note on silicon in rice endosperm. *Cereal Chem.*, 52: 854-856.

Khan, M.A. & Eggum, B.O. 1978. Effect of baking on the nutritive value of Pakistani bread. *J. Sci. Food Agric.*, 29: 1069-1075.

Khan, M.A. & Eggum, B.O. 1979. Effect of home and industrial processing on protein quality of baby foods and breakfast cereals. *J. Sci. Food Agric.*, 30: 369-376.

Khandker, A.K., de Mosqueda, M.B., del Rosario, R.R. & Juliano, B.O. 1986. Factors affecting properties of rice noodles prepared with an extruder. *ASEAN Food J.*, 2: 31-35.

Khin-Maung-U, Bolin, T.D., Pereira, S.P., Duncombe, V.M., Nyunt-Nyunt-Wai, Myo-Khin & Linklater, J.M. 1990a. Absorption of carbohydrate from rice in Burmese village children and adults. *Am. J. Clin. Nutr.*, 52: 342-347.

Khin-Maung-U, Pereira, S.P., Bolin, T.D., Duncombe, V.M., Myo-Khin, Nyunt-Nyunt-Wai & Linklater, J.M. 1990b. Malabsorption of carbohydrate from rice and child growth: a longitudinal study with the breath-hydrogen test in Burmese village children and adults. *Am. J. Clin. Nutr.*, 52: 348-352.

Khor, G.L., Tee, E.S. & Kandiah, M. 1990. Patterns of food production and consumption in the ASEAN Region. *World Rev. Nutr. Diet.*, 61: 1-40.

Khush, G.S. & Juliano, B.O. 1985. Breeding for high-yielding rices of excellent cooking and eating qualities. In *Rice grain quality and marketing*, p. 61-69. Manila, IRRI.

Kik, M.C. & Williams, R.R. 1945. *The nutritional improvement of white rice.* Nat. Acad. Sci. Bull. 112. Washington, D.C., National Research Council. 76 pp.

Kitagishi, K. & Yamane, I., eds. 1981. *Heavy metal pollution in soils in Japan.* Tokyo, Japan Scientific Societies Press. 302 pp.

Kondo, H., Abe, K. & Arai, S. 1989. Immunoassay of oryzacystatin occurring in rice seeds during maturation and germination. *Agric. Biol. Chem.*, 53: 2949-2954.

Kumamaru, T., Satoh, H., Iwata, N., Omura, T., Ogawa, M. & Tanaka, K. 1988. Mutants of rice storage proteins. 1. Screening of mutants for rice storage proteins of protein bodies in the starchy endosperm. *Theor. Appl. Genet.*, 76: 11-16.

Kumar, I. & Khush, G.S. 1987. Genetic analysis of different amylose levels in rice. *Crop Sci.*, 27: 1167-1172.

Kumar, I., Khush, G.S. & Juliano, B.O. 1987. Genetic analysis of *waxy* locus in rice (*Oryza sativa* L.). *Theor. Appl. Genet.*, 73: 481-488.

Kunze, O.R. 1985. Effect of environment and variety on milling qualities of rice. In *Rice grain quality and marketing*, p. 37-47. Manila, IRRI.

Kunze, O.R. & Calderwood, D.L. 1985. Rough rice drying. *In* B.O. Juliano, ed. *Rice chemistry and technology*, 2nd ed., p. 233-263. St Paul, MN, USA, Am. Assoc. Cereal Chem.

Lai, M.-N., Chang, W.T.H. & Luh, B.S. 1980. Rice vinegar fermentation. *In* B.S. Luh, ed. *Rice: production and utilization*, p. 690-711. Westport, CT, USA, AVI Publishing Co.

Levitt, M.D., Hirsch, P., Fetzer, C.A., Sheahan, M. & Levine, A.S. 1987. H$_2$ excretion after ingestion of complex carbohydrates. *Gastroenterology*, 92: 383-389.

Li, B.-J. & Lai, L.-Z. 1989. The study on the breeding of "black superior rice" by using biotechniques. *Proc. 6th Int. Congr. SABRAO*, p. 289-291.

Li, C.-F. & Luh, B.S. 1980. Rice snack foods. *In* B.S. Luh, ed. *Rice: production and utilization*, p. 690-711.

Westport, CT, USA, AVI Publishing Co.

Lin, T.-C., Shao, Y.-Y. & Chiang, W. 1988. Investigation of the processing and the quality of rice milk. *J. Chin. Agric. Chem. Soc.*, 26: 130-137.

Little, R.R., Hilder, G.B. & Dawson, E.H. 1958. Differential effect of dilute alkali on 25 varieties of milled white rice. *Cereal Chem.*, 35: 111-126.

Liu, J.-X., Lu, Z.-H. & Su, Q. 1985. Regional selenium deficiency of feedstuffs in China. *Sci. Agric. Sin.*, 1985(4): 76-79.

Livesey, G. 1990. The energy values of unavailable carbohydrates and diets. An enquiry and analysis. *Am. J. Clin. Nutr.*, 51: 617-637.

Lopez de Romaña, G., Graham, G.G., Mellits, E.D. & MacLean, W.C. Jr. 1980. Utilization of the protein and energy of the potato by human infants. *J. Nutr.*, 110: 1849-1857.

Lu, J.J. & Chang, T.T. 1980. Rice in its temporal and spatial perspective. *In* B.S. Luh, ed. *Rice: production and utilization*, p. 1-74. Westport, CT, USA, AVI Publishing Co.

Luh, B.S., ed. 1980. *Rice: production and utilization*. Westport, CT, USA, AVI Publishing Co. 925 pp.

Luh, B.S. & Bhumiratana, A. 1980. Breakfast rice cereals and baby foods. *In* B.S. Luh, ed. *Rice: production and utilization*, p. 622-649. Westport, CT, USA, AVI Publishing Co.

MacLean, W.C. Jr, Klein, G.L., Lopez de Romaña, G., Massa, E. & Graham, G.G. 1978. Protein quality of conventional and high-protein rice and digestibility of glutinous and nonglutinous rice by preschool children. *J. Nutr.*, 108: 1740-1747.

MacLean, W.C. Jr, Lopez de Romaña, G., Klein, G.L., Massa, E., Mellits, E.D. & Graham, G.G. 1979. Digestibility and utilization of the energy and protein of wheat by infants. *J. Nutr.*, 109: 1290-1298.

MacLean, W.C. Jr, Lopez de Romaña, G., Placko, R.P. & Graham, G.G. 1981. Protein quality and digestibility of sorghum in preschool children: balance studies and plasma free amino acid. *J. Nutr.*, 111: 1928-1936.

MacRitchie, F., du Cros, D.L. & Wrigley, C.W. 1990. Flour polypeptides related to wheat quality. *Adv. Cereal Sci. Technol.*, 10: 79-145.

Maneepun, S. 1987. Production and consumption of processed rice products in Thailand. In *Proceedings,*

International Symposium Dietary Life of Rice-Eating Populations, Kyoto, 24 October 1987, p. 33-40. Kyoto, Research Institute for Product Development.

Marfo, E.K., Simpson, B.K., Idowre, J.S. & Oke, O.L. 1990. Effect of local food processing on phytate levels in cassava, cocoyam, yam, maize, sorghum, rice, cowpea and soybean. *J. Agric. Food Chem.*, 38: 1580-1585.

Matsuda, T., Sugiyama, M., Nakamura, R. & Torii, S. 1988. Purification and properties of an allergenic protein in rice grain. *Agric. Biol. Chem.*, 52: 1465-1470.

Miao, G.-H. & Tang, X.-H. 1986. Isolation, purification and the properties of rice germ lectin receptors in rice embryo and endosperm. *Kexue Tongbao* (Engl. transl.), 22: 1569-1573.

Mickus, R.R. & Luh, B.S. 1980. Rice enrichment with vitamins and amino acids. *In* B.S. Luh, ed. *Rice: production and utilization*, p. 486-500. Westport, CT, USA, AVI Publishing Co.

Misaki, M. & Yasumatsu, K. 1985. Rice enrichment and fortification. *In* B.O. Juliano, ed. *Rice chemistry and technology*, 2nd ed., p. 389-401. St Paul, MN, USA, Am. Assoc. Cereal Chem.

Mitchell, C.R., Mitchell, P.R. & Nissenbaum, R. 1988. *Nutritional rice milk production.* U.S. Patent No. 4,744,992. 8 pp.

Miyoshi, H., Okuda, T., Kobayashi, N., Okuda K. & Koishi, H. 1987a. Effects of rice fiber on mineral balance in young Japanese men. *Nippon Eiyo Shokuryo Gakkaishi*, 40: 165-170 (in Japanese).

Miyoshi, H., Okuda, T. & Koishi, H. 1988. Effects of feeding of polished rice, brown rice and rice bran on digestibility of nutrients by growing rats. *Sci. Living Annu. Rep., Osaka City Univ.*, 36: 7-11 (in Japanese).

Miyoshi, H., Okuda, T., Oi, Y. & Koishi, H. 1986. Effect of rice fiber on fecal weight, apparent digestibility of energy, nitrogen and fat and degradation of neutral detergent fiber in young men. *J. Nutr. Sci. Vitaminol.*, 32: 581-589.

Miyoshi, H., Okuda, T., Okuda, K. & Koishi, H. 1987b. Effect of brown rice on apparent digestibility and balance of nutrients in young men on low protein diets. *J. Nutr. Sci. Vitaminol.*, 33: 207-218.

Molla, A.M., Ahmed, S.M. & Greenough, W.B. III. 1985. Rice-based oral rehydration solution decreases the stool volume in acute diarrhea. *Bull. WHO*, 63: 751-756.

Morishita, T., Fumoto, N., Yoshizawa, T. & Kagawa, K. 1987. Varietal differences in cadmium levels of rice grains of japonica, indica, javanica, and hybrid varieties produced in the same plot of a field. *Soil Sci. Plant Nutr.*, 33: 629-637.

Mossé, J. 1990. Nitrogen to protein conversion factors for ten cereals and six legumes or oilseeds. A reappraisal of its definition and determination. Variation according to species and to seed protein content. *J. Agric. Food Chem.*, 38: 18-24.

Mossé, J., Huet, J.-C. & Baudet, J. 1988. The amino acid composition of rice grain as a function of nitrogen content as compared to other cereals: a reappraisal of rice chemical scores. *J. Cereal Sci.*, 8: 165-175.

Mossman, A.P. 1986. A review of basic concepts in rice-drying research. *Crit. Rev. Food Sci. Nutr.*, 25: 49-71.

Murata, K., Kitagawa, T. & Juliano, B.O. 1978. Protein quality of high protein rice in rats. *Agric. Biol. Chem.*, 42: 565-570.

Murugesan, G. & Bhattacharya, K.R. 1991. Basis for varietal difference in popping expansion of rice. *J. Cereal Sci.*, 13: 71-83.

Nicolosi, R. 1990. Unsaponifiables in rice bran oil under study. *Int. News Fats Oils Rel. Mater. (INFORM)* 1: 831-832, 834-835.

Nielsen, H.K., De Weck, D., Finot, P.A., Liardon, R. & Hurrell, R.F. 1985. Stability of tryptophan during food processing and storage. I. Comparative losses of tryptophan, lysine and methionine in different model systems. *Br. J. Nutr.*, 53: 281-292.

Nikuni, Z., Hizukuri, S., Kumagai, K., Hasegawa, H., Moriwaki, T., Fukui, T., Doi, K., Nara, S. & Maeda, I. 1969. The effect of temperature during the maturation period on the physico-chemical properties of potato and rice starches. *Mem. Inst. Sci. Ind. Res. Osaka Univ.*, 26: 1-27.

Noda, K., Hirai, S. & Dambara, H. 1987. Selenium content of brown rice grown in Japan. *Agric. Biol. Chem.*, 51: 2451-2455.

Normand, F.L., Ory, R.L. & Mod, R.R. 1981. Interactions of several bile acids with hemicelluloses from several varieties of rice. *J. Food Sci.*, 46: 1159-1161.

Normand, F.L., Ory, R.L., Mod, R.R., Saunders, R.M. & Gumbmann, M.R. 1984. Influence of rice hemicellulose and α-cellulose on lipid and water content of rice faeces and on blood lipids. *J. Cereal Sci.*, 2: 37-42.

Obata, Y. & Tanaka, H. 1965. Studies on the photolysis of ʟ-cysteine and ʟ-cystine. Formation of the flavor of cooked rice from ʟ-cysteine and ʟ-cystine. *Agric. Biol. Chem.*, 29: 191-195.

Ogawa, M., Kumamaru, T., Satoh, H., Iwata, N., Omura, T., Kasai, Z. & Tanaka, K. 1987. Purification of protein body-I of rice seed and its polypeptide composition. *Plant Cell Physiol.*, 28: 1517-1527.

Ogawa, M., Kumamaru, T., Satoh, H., Omura, T., Park, T., Shintaku, K. & Baba, K. 1989. Mutants of rice storage proteins. 2. Isolation and characterization of protein bodies from rice mutants. *Theor. Appl. Genet.*, 78: 305-310.

Ogawa, M., Tanaka, K. & Kasai, Z. 1977. Note on the phytin-containing particles isolated from rice scutellum. *Cereal Chem.*, 54: 1029-1034.

Ohta, H., Aibara, S., Yamashita, H., Sekiyama, F. & Morita, Y. 1990. Post-harvest drying of fresh rice grain and its effects on deterioration of lipids during storage. *Agric. Biol. Chem.*, 54: 1157-1164.

Omura, T. & Satoh, H. 1984. Mutation of grain properties in rice. *In* S. Tsunoda & N. Takahashi, eds. *Biology of rice*, p. 293-303. Tokyo, Japan Scientific Societies Press; Amsterdam, Elsevier.

Ory, R.L., Bog-Hansen, T.C. & Mod, R.R. 1981. Properties of hemagglutinins in rice and other cereal grains. *In* R.L. Ory, ed. *Antinutrients and natural toxicants in foods*. Westport, CT, USA, Food & Nutrition Press.

Padua, A.B. & Juliano, B.O. 1974. Effect of parboiling on thiamin, protein and fat of rice. *J. Sci. Food Agric.*, 25: 697-701.

Palmiano, E.P. & Juliano, B.O. 1972. Physicochemical properties of Niigata waxy rices. *Agric. Biol. Chem.*, 36: 157-159.

Panlasigui, L.N. 1989. *Glycemic response to rice*. Ph.D. dissertation, University of Toronto, Department of Nutritional Sciences. 171 pp.

Pedersen, B. & Eggum, B.O. 1983. The influence of milling on the nutritive value of flour from cereal grains. IV. Rice. *Qual. Plant. Plant Foods Hum. Nutr.*, 33: 267-278.

Pereira, S.M., Begum, A. & Juliano, B.O. 1981. Effect of high protein rice on nitrogen retention and growth of preschool children on a rice-based diet. *Qual. Plant. Plant Foods Hum. Nutr.*, 31: 97-108.

Perez, C.M., Cagampang, G.B., Esmama, B.V., Monserrate, R.U. & Juliano, B.O. 1973. Protein metabolism in leaves and developing grains of rices differing in grain protein content. *Plant Physiol.*, 51: 537-542.

Perez, C.M. & Juliano, B.O. 1988. Varietal differences in quality characteristics of rice layer cakes and fermented cakes. *Cereal Chem.*, 65: 40-43.

Perez, C.M., Juliano, B.O., Pascual, C.G. & Novenario, V.G 1987. Extracted lipids and carbohydrates during washing and boiling of milled rice. *Starch*, 39: 386-390.

Pillaiyar, P. 1988. *Rice postproduction manual.* New Delhi, Wiley Eastern Ltd. 437 pp.

Poola, I. 1989. Rice lectin: physicochemical and carbohydrate-binding properties. *Carbohydr. Polym.*, 10: 281-288.

Raghuram, T.C., Brahmaji Rao, U. & Rukmini, C. 1989. Studies on hypolipidemic effects of dietary rice bran oil in human subjects. *Nutr. Rep. Int.*, 39: 889-895.

Rand, W.M., Uauy, R. & Scrimshaw, N.S., eds. 1984. *Protein-energy-requirement studies in developing countries: results of international research. UN Univ. Food Nutr. Bull. Suppl.,* Vol. 10. 369 pp.

Reeck, G.R., Muthukrishnan, S. & Kramer, K.J. 1990. Cereal inhibitors of insect amylases and sulfhydryl proteases. *Abstracts 4th Annual Meeting, Rockefeller Foundation's International Program on Rice Biotechnology,* IRRI, 9-12 May 1990. New York, Rockefeller Foundation.

Rehana, F., Basappa, S.C. & Sreenivasa Murthy, V. 1979. Destruction of aflatoxin in rice by different cooking methods. *J. Food Sci. Technol.*, 16: 111-112.

Reilly, A. 1990. Grain quality as affected by microorganisms in tropical regions. *Food Lab. News,* 21: 32-35.

Resurrección, A.P., Hara, T., Juliano, B.O. & Yoshida, S. 1977. Effect of temperature during ripening on grain quality of rice. *Soil Sci. Plant Nutr.*, 23: 109-112.

Resurrección, A.P. & Juliano, B.O. 1981. Properties of poorly digestible fraction of protein bodies of cooked milled rice. *Qual. Plant. Plant Foods Hum. Nutr.*, 31: 119-128.

Resurrección, A.P., Juliano, B.O. & Eggum, B.O. 1978. Preparation and properties of destarched milled rice. *Nutr. Rep. Int.*, 18: 17-25.

Resurrección, A.P., Juliano, B.O. & Tanaka, Y. 1979. Nutrient content and distribution in milling fractions of rice grain. *J. Sci. Food Agric.*, 30: 475-481.

Resurrección, A.P., Li, X.S., Okita, T.W. & Juliano, B.O. 1992. Characterization of poorly digested protein of cooked rice protein bodies. *Cereal Chem.* (in press).

Rivai, I.F., Koyama, H. & Suzuki, S. 1990. Cadmium content of rice and its daily intake in various countries. *Bull. Environ. Contam. Toxicol.*, 44: 910-916.

Rivera, E.F., Aligui, G.L., Taaca, A., Juliano, B.O. & Perez, C.M. 1983. The use of "am" (rice water) among cases of acute gastroenteritis in children. *Philipp. J. Pediatr.*, 32: 22-29.

Robert, L.S., Thompson, R.D. & Flavell, R.B. 1989. Tissue-specific expression of a wheat high molecular weight glutenin gene in transgenic tobacco. *Plant Cell*, 1: 569-578.

Roberts, R.L. 1972. Quick-cooking rice. *In* D.F. Houston, ed. *Rice chemistry and technology*, p. 381-399. St Paul, MN, USA, Am. Assoc. Cereal Chem.

Roxas, B.V., Intengan, C.Ll. & Juliano, B.O. 1975. Effect of protein content of milled rice on nitrogen retention of Filipino children fed a rice-fish diet. *Nutr. Rep. Int.*, 11: 393-398.

Roxas, B.V., Intengan, C.Ll. & Juliano, B.O. 1976. Protein content of milled rice and nitrogen retention of preschool children fed rice-mung bean diets. *Nutr. Rep. Int.*, 14: 203-207.

Roxas, B.V., Intengan, C.Ll. & Juliano, B.O. 1979. Protein quality of high-protein and low-protein milled rices in preschool children. *J. Nutr.*, 109: 832-839.

Roxas, B.V., Intengan, C.Ll. & Juliano, B.O. 1980. Effect of zinc supplementation and high-protein rice on the growth of preschool children on a rice-based diet. *Qual. Plant. Plant Foods Hum. Nutr.*, 30: 213-222.

Roxas, B.V., Loyola, A.S. & Reyes, E.L. 1978. The effect of different degrees of rice milling on nitrogen digestibility and retention. *Philipp. J. Nutr.*, 31: 110-113.

Russell, P.L., Berry, C.S. & Greenwell, P. 1989. Characterization of resistant starch from wheat and maize. *J. Cereal Sci.*, 9: 1-15.

Sagara, Y. 1988. The rice surplus, and new technology for rice processing in Japan. *Food Fert. Technol. Cent. Asian Pac. Reg. Ext. Bull.*, 273: 11-27.

Salcedo, J. Jr, Bamba, M.D., Carrasco, E.O., Chan, G.S., Concepcion, I., Jose, F.R., de Leon, J.F., Oliveros, S.B., Pascual, C.R.,

Santiago, L.C. & Valenzuela, R.C. 1950. Artificial enrichment of white rice as a solution to endemic beriberi. Report of field trials in Bataan, Philippines. *J. Nutr.*, 42: 501-523.

Sanchez, P.C., Juliano, B.O., Laude, V.T. & Perez, C.M. 1988. Nonwaxy rice for *tapuy* (rice wine) production. *Cereal Chem.*, 65: 240-243.

Sanchez, P.C., Laude, V.T., Yap, A.B., & Juliano, B.O. 1989. Effect of toasting and variety on "tapuy" quality. *Philipp. Agric.*, 72: 225-230.

Santiago, M.I.C., Roxas, B.V., Intengan, C.Ll. & Juliano, B.O. 1984. Protein and energy utilization of brown, undermilled and milled rices by preschool children. *Qual. Plant. Plant Foods Hum. Nutr.*, 34: 15-25.

Satin, M. 1988. Bread without wheat. *In* S. Maneepun, P. Varangoon & B. Phithakpol, eds. *Food science and technology in industrial development. Proceedings Foods Conference '88*, Bangkok, 24-26 October 1988, Vol. 1, p. 42-47. Bangkok, Kasetsart University Institute of Food Research & Product Development.

Saunders, R.M. 1990. The properties of rice bran as a foodstuff. *Cereal Foods World*, 35: 632, 634-636.

Schaeffer, G.W. & Sharpe, F.T. Jr. 1983. Improved rice proteins in plants regenerated from S-AEC-resistant callus. In *Proceedings of a Workshop on Cell and Tissue Culture Techniques for Cereal Crop Improvement,* Beijing, 1981, p. 279-290. Beijing, Science Press; Manila, IRRI.

Scrimshaw, N.S. 1988. Nutrition and health — new knowledge, new challenges. *In* K. Yasumoto, Y. Itokawa, H. Koishi & Y. Sanno, eds. *Proceedings, 5th Asian Congress Nutrition*, Osaka, 26-29 October 1987, p. 6-23. Tokyo, Center for Academic Publications Japan.

Seiber, J.M., Heinrichs, E.A., Aquino, G.B., Valencia, S.L., Andrade, P. & Argente, A.M. 1978. *Residues of carbofuran applied as a systematic insecticide in irrigated wetland rice — implications for insect control.* IRRI Research Paper Ser. 17. Manila, IRRI. 27 pp.

Seshu, D.V., Krishnasamy, V. & Siddique, S.B. 1988. Seed vigor in rice. In *Rice seed health. Proceedings of IRRI/UNDP International Workshop*, IRRI, 16-20 March 1987, p. 315-329. Manila, IRRI.

Shankara, T., Ananthachar, T.K., Narasimha, V., Krishnamurthy, H. & Desikachar, H.S.R. 1984. Improvements of the traditional edge runner process for rice flake production. *J. Food Sci. Technol.*, 21: 121-122.

Sharma, R.D. & Rukmini, C. 1986. Rice bran oil and hypocholesterolemia in rats. *Lipids*, 21: 715-717.

Sharma, R.D. & Rukmini, C. 1987. Hypocholesterolemic activity of unsaponifiable matter of rice bran oil. *Indian J. Med. Res.*, 85: 278-281.

Shibuya, N. 1989. Comparative studies on the cell wall polymers obtained from different parts of rice grains. *In* N.G. Lewis & M.G. Paice, eds. *Plant cell wall polymers: biogenesis and biodegradation*, Symp. No. 399, p. 333-344. Washington, D.C., Am. Chem. Soc.

Siscar-Lee, J.J.H., Juliano, B.O., Qureshi, R.H. & Akbar, M. 1990. Effect of saline soil on grain quality of rices differing in salinity tolerance. *Plant Foods Hum. Nutr.*, 40: 31-36.

Soni, S.K. & Sandhu, D.K. 1989. Fermentation of *idli*: effects of changes in raw materials and physico-chemical conditions. *J. Cereal Sci.*, 10: 227-238.

Sosulski, F.W. & Imafidon, G.I. 1990. Amino acid composition and nitrogen-to-protein conversion factors for animal and plant foods. *J. Agric. Food Chem.*, 38: 1351-1356.

Souci, S.W., Fuchmann, W. & Kraut, H. 1986. *Food composition and nutrition tables 1986/87*, 3rd rev. ed. Stuttgart, Wissenschaftliche Verlagsgesellschaft mbH.

Sowbhagya, C.M. & Bhattacharya, K.R. 1976. Lipid autoxidation in rice. *J. Food Sci.*, 41: 1018-1023.

Srinivas, T. & Bhashyam, M.K. 1985. Effect of variety and environment on milling quality of rice. In *Rice grain quality and marketing*, p. 51-59. Manila, IRRI.

Srinivas, T. & Desikachar, H.S.R. 1973. Factors affecting the puffing quality of paddy. *J. Sci. Food Agric.*, 24: 883-891.

Srinivasa Rao, P. 1970. Studies on the nature of carbohydrate moiety in high yielding varieties of rice. *J. Nutr.*, 101: 879-884.

Srinivasa Rao, P. 1976. Nature of carbohydrates in red rice varieties. *Plant Foods Man*, 2: 69-74.

Steinkraus, K.H., ed. 1983. *Handbook of indigenous fermented foods*. New York, Marcel Dekker, Inc. 671 pp.

Stemmermann, G.N. & Kolonel, L.N. 1978. Talc-coated rice as a risk factor for stomach cancer. *Am. J. Clin. Nutr.*, 31: 2017-2019.

Stucy Johnson, F.C. 1988. Utilization of American-produced rice in muffins for gluten-sensitive individuals. *Home Econ. Res. J.*, 17: 175-183.

Sugimoto, T., Tanaka, K. & Kasai, Z. 1986. Molecular species in the protein body II (PB-II) of developing rice endosperm. *Agric. Biol. Chem.*, 50: 3031-3035.

Susheelamma, N.S. & Rao, M.V.L. 1979. Functional role of the arabinogalactan of black gram (*Phaseolus mungo*) in the texture of leavened foods (steamed puddings). *J. Food Sci.*, 44: 1309-1312, 1316.

Suzuki, S., Tetsuka, T., Kajiwara, K. & Mitani, M. 1962. Influence of several lipids on human serum cholesterol. V. Effect of rice oil. *Jpn. J. Nutr.*, 20: 139-141 (in Japanese).

Taira, H., Nakagahra, M. & Nagamine, T. 1988. Fatty acid composition of indica, sinica, japonica, and japonica groups of nonglutinous brown rice. *J. Agric. Food Chem.*, 36: 45-47.

Taira, H., Taira, H. & Fujii, K. 1979. Influence of cropping season on lipid content and fatty acid composition of lowland nonglutinous brown rice. *Nippon Sakumotsu Gakkai Kiji*, 48: 371-377.

Takahashi, K., Sugimoto, T., Miura, T., Wasizu, Y. & Yoshizawa, K. 1989. Isolation and identification of red rice pigments. *Nippon Jozo Kyokai Zasshi*, 84: 807-812.

Takeda, Y., Hizukuri, S. & Juliano, B.O. 1987. Structures of rice amylopectin with low and high affinities for iodine. *Carbohydr. Res.*, 168: 79-88.

Tanaka, K. & Ogawa, M. 1988. Storage protein genes and their expression control: specially focusing on the improvement of PB-I digestibility. *Abstracts Annual Meeting Rockefeller Foundation Program on Rice Biotechnology*, IRRI, 20-22 January 1988. Manila, IRRI.

Tanaka, K., Ogawa, M. & Kasai, Z. 1977. The rice scutellum. II. A comparison of scutellar and aleurone electron-dense particles by transmission electron microscopy including energy-dispersive X-ray analysis. *Cereal Chem.*, 54: 684-689.

Tanaka, K., Sugimoto, T., Ogawa, M. & Kasai, Z. 1980. Isolation and characterization of two types of protein bodies in the rice endosperm. *Agric. Biol. Chem.*, 44: 1633-1639.

Tanaka, K., Yoshida, T., Asada, K. & Kasai, Z. 1973. Subcellular particles isolated from aleurone layer of rice seeds. *Arch. Biochem. Biophys.*, 155: 136-143.

Tanaka, Y., Hayashida, S. & Hongo, M. 1975. Quantitative relation between feces protein particles and rice protein bodies. *Nippon Nogei Kagaku Kaishi*, 49: 425-429.

Tanaka, Y., Resurrección, A.P., Juliano, B.O. & Bechtel, D.B 1978. Properties of whole and undigested fraction of protein bodies of milled rice. *Agric. Biol. Chem.*, 42: 2015-2023.

Tanchoco, C.C., Castro, M.C.A., Alcaraz, S.A., Bassig, M.C.C., de los Santos, E. & Lana, R.D. 1990. *Glycemic effects of different sources and forms of carbohydrate foods and levels of fiber.* Paper presented at the Food Nutr. Res. Inst. 16th Seminar Ser., Manila, 19-20 July.

Tang, S.X., Khush, G.S. & Juliano, B.O. 1989. Diallel analysis of gel consistency in rice (*Oryza sativa* L.). *SABRAO J.*, 21: 135-142.

Tani, T. 1985. Rice processing industries in Japan. In *FAO/UNDP Regional Workshop on Rice Processing Industries,* Jakarta, 15-20 July, p. 88-101. Bangkok, FAO Regional Office for Asia and the Pacific.

Tanphaichitr, V. 1985. Epidemiology and clinical assessment of vitamin deficiencies in Thai children. *In* R.E. Eeckels, O. Ransome-Kuti & C.C. Kroonenberg, eds. *Child health in the tropics*, p. 151-166. Dordrecht, the Netherlands, M. Nijhoff Publishers.

Toenniessen, G.H. & Herdt, R.W. 1989. The Rockefeller Foundation's international program on rice biotechnology. *In* J.I. Cohen, ed. *Strengthening collaboration in biotechnology: international agricultural research and the private sector,* p. 291-317. Washington, D.C., US Agency for International Development, Bureau for Science and Technology.

Tontisirin, K., Ajmanwra, N. & Valyasevi, A. 1984. Long-term study on the adequacy of usual Thai weaning food for young children. *UN Univ. Food Nutr. Bull. Suppl.*, 10: 265-285.

Tontisirin, K., Sirichakawal, P.P. & Valyasevi, A. 1981. Protein requirements of adult Thai males. *UN Univ. Food Nutr. Bull. Suppl.*, 5: 88-97.

Topping, D.L., Illman, R.J., Roach, P.D., Trimble, R.P., Kambouris, A. & Nestel, P.J. 1990. Modulation of the hypolipidemic effect of fish oils by dietary fiber in fats: studies with rice and wheat bran. *J. Nutr.*, 120: 325-330.

Torún, B., Young, V. R. & Rand, W. R., eds. 1981. *Protein-energy requirements of developing countries: evaluation of new data. UN Univ. Food Nutr. Bull. Suppl.*, Vol. 5. 268 pp.

Tribelhorn, R.E., O'Deen, L.A., Harper, J.M. & Fellers, D.A. 1986. *Investigation on extrusion for ORT samples.* Boulder, CO, USA, Colorado State University Research Foundation. 70 pp.

Trowell, H. 1987. Diabetes mellitus and rice — a hypothesis. *Human Nutr.: Food Sci. Nutr.,* 41F: 145-152.

Tsai, S.T., Chwang, L.C., Doong, T.I. & Mu, H.L. 1990. Glycemic response of rice and rice products in NIDDM. In *Program and abstracts, Asian Symposium on Rice and Nutrition,* Taipei, 22-23 June 1990, p. 54. Taipei, Taipei Dietitians Association.

Tsugita, T. 1986. Aroma of cooked rice. *Food Rev. Int.,* 1: 497-520.

Tsutsumi, C. & Shimomura, C. 1978. Changes of the contents of mineral elements and protein by milling and washing with water. *Shokuhin Sogo Kenkyusho Kenkyu Hokoku,* 33: 12-17.

Tulpule, P.G., Nagarajan, V. & Bhat, R.V. 1982. *Environment causes of food contamination.* Environment India Review — Series 1. New Delhi, Government of India, Department of Environment.

UNICEF. 1991. *State of the world's children.* New York, UNICEF.

United Nations. 1987. *First report on the world nutrition situation.* Rome, FAO Administrative Committee on Coordination, Subcommittee on Nutrition.

Unnevehr, L.J., Juliano, B.O., Perez, C.M. & Marciano, E.B. 1985. *Consumer demand for rice grain quality in Thailand, Indonesia, and the Philippines.* IRRI Research Paper Ser. 116. Manila, IRRI. 20 pp.

Unnevehr, L.J. & Stanford, M.L. 1985. Technology and the demand for women's labour in Asian rice farming. In *Women in rice farming,* p. 1-20. Aldershot, Hants., UK, Gower Publishing Co. Ltd.

van Ruiten, H.T.L. 1985. Rice milling: an overview. *In* B.O. Juliano, ed. *Rice chemistry and technology,* 2nd ed., p. 349-388. St Paul, MN, USA, Am. Assoc. Cereal Chem.

Vasanthi, S. & Bhat, R.V. 1990. Aflatoxins in stored rice. *Int. Rice Res. Newsl.,* 15(1): 39-40.

Ventura, B. 1977. Rice bran utilization in the prevention and treatment of dental decay (caries). In *Proceedings. Rice By-products Utilization International Conference,* Valencia, 1974, Vol. 4, *Rice bran utilization: food and feed,* p. 215-218. Valencia, Instituto de Agroquimica y Tecnologia de Alimentos.

Vijayagopal, P. & Kurup, P.A. 1972. Hypolipidaemic activity of whole paddy in rats fed a high-fat high-cholesterol diet. Isolation of an active fraction from the husk and bran. *Atherosclerosis*, 15: 215-222.

Villareal, C.P. & Juliano, B.O. 1987. Varietal differences in quality characteristics of puffed rice. *Cereal Chem.*, 64: 337-342.

Villareal, C.P. & Juliano, B.O. 1989a. Variability in contents of thiamine and riboflavin in brown rice, crude oil in brown rice and bran-polish, and silicon in hull of IR rices. *Plant Foods Hum. Nutr.*, 39: 287-297.

Villareal, C.P. & Juliano, B.O. 1989b. Comparative level of waxy gene product of endosperm starch granules of different rice ecotypes. *Starch*, 41: 369-371.

Villareal, C.P., Juliano, B.O. & Sauphanor, B. 1990. Grain quality of rices grown in irrigated and upland cultures. *Plant Foods Hum. Nutr.*, 40: 37-47.

Villareal, C.P., Maranville, J.W. & Juliano, B.O. 1991. Nutrient content and retention during milling of brown rices from the International Rice Research Institute. *Cereal Chem.*, 68: 437-439.

Villareal, R.M. & Juliano, B.O. 1978. Properties of glutelin from mature and developing rice grain. *Phytochemistry*, 17: 177-182.

Wang, H.-H. 1980. Fermented rice products. *In* B.S. Luh, ed. *Rice: production and utilization*, p. 650-689. Westport, CT, USA, AVI Publishing Co.

Watanabe, M., Miyakawa, J., Ikezawa, Z., Suzuki, Y., Hirao, T., Yoshizawa, T. & Arai, S. 1990a. Production of hypoallergenic rice by enzymatic decomposition of constituent proteins. *J. Food Sci.*, 55: 781-783.

Watanabe, M., Yoshizawa, T., Miyakawa, J., Ikezawa, Z., Abe, K., Yanagesawa, T. & Arai, S. 1990b. Quality improvement and evaluation of hypoallergenic rice grains. *J. Food Sci.*, 55: 1105-1107.

Watt, B.K. & Merrill, A.L. 1963. *Composition of foods*. Agric. Handbook 8. Washington, D.C., US Dept. Agric. Consumer and Food Economics Res. Div. 190 pp.

WHO. 1985. *Energy and protein requirements. Report of a Joint FAO/WHO/UNU Expert Consultation.* WHO Tech. Rep. Ser. 724. Geneva, WHO. 206 pp.

Williams, R.R. 1956. *Williams-Waterman Fund for the Combat of Dietary Diseases. A history of the period 1935 through 1955.* New York, Research Corporation. 120 pp.

Wolever, T.M.S., Jenkins, D.J.A., Kalmusky, J., Jenkins, A.,

Giordano, C., Guidici, S., Josse, R.G. & Wong, G.S. 1986. Comparison of regular and parboiled rices: explanation of discrepancies between reported glycemic responses to rice. *Nutr. Res.,* 6: 349-357.

Wong, H.B. 1981. Rice water in treatment of infantile gastroenteritis. *Lancet,* (2): 102-103.

Yamagata, H., Sugimoto, T., Tanaka, K. & Kasai, Z. 1982. Biosynthesis of storage proteins in developing rice seeds. *Plant Physiol.,* 70: 1094-1100.

Yap, A.B., Ilag, L.L., Juliano, B.O. & Perez, C.M. 1987. Soaking in *Aspergillus parasiticus*-inoculated water and aflatoxin in parboiled rice. *Hum. Nutr.: Food Sci. Nutr.,* 41F: 225-229.

Yap, A.B., Perez, C.M. & Juliano, B.O. 1990. Artificial yellowing of rice at 60ºC. *In* J.O. Naewbanij, ed. *Advances in grain postharvest technology generation and utilization. Proceedings 11th ASEAN Technical Seminar on Grain Postharvest Technology,* Kuala Lumpur, 23-26 August 1988, p. 3-20. Bangkok, ASEAN Crops Postharvest Programme.

Yokoo, M. 1990. Producing new rice (Super-rice program). *Farming Jpn.,* 24(1): 29-40.

Yoshida, S. 1981. *Fundamentals of rice crop science.* Los Baños, Laguna, the Philippines, IRRI.

Yoshizawa, K. & Kishi, S. 1985. Rice in brewing. *In* B.O. Juliano, ed. *Rice chemistry and technology,* 2nd ed., p. 619-645. St Paul, MN, USA, Am. Assoc. Cereal Chem.